THE COMPLETE SELF HEALING COLLECTION OF

DR. SEBI'S

NATURAL HERBAL REMEDIES

Everything You Need to Know to Restore Your Body's Ability to Heal Itself and Live a Disease-Free Life

Emily Carter

Copyright 2025 – Emily Carter © All rights reserved.

The content contained within this book may not be reproduced, duplicated, or transmitted without direct written permission from the author or the publisher. Under no circumstances will any blame or legal responsibility be held against the publisher, or author, for any damages, reparation, or monetary loss due to the information contained within this book. Either directly or indirectly.

Legal Notice:

This book is copyright protected. This book is only for personal use. You cannot amend, distribute, sell, use, quote or paraphrase any part, or the content within this book, without the consent of the author or publisher.

Disclaimer Notice:

Please note the information contained within this document is for educational and entertainment purposes only. All effort has been executed to present accurate, up to date, and reliable, complete information. No warranties of any kind are declared or implied. Readers acknowledge that the author is not engaging in the rendering of legal, financial, medical, or professional advice. The content within this book has been derived from various sources. Please consult a licensed professional before attempting any techniques outlined in this book.

By reading this document, the reader agrees that under no circumstances is the author responsible for any losses, direct or indirect, which are incurred because of the use of information contained within this document, including, but not limited to, errors, omissions, or inaccuracies.

Table of Contents

DON'T MISS THIS! 7
   The Self-Healing Bonus Bundle You'll Wish You Had Sooner... 7

INTRODUCTION 8

CHAPTER 1: WHO WAS DR. SEBI? 10
   THE CONCEPT OF INTRACELLULAR CLEANING 10
   THE ROLE OF MUCUS AND THE LINK TO DISEASE 11
      Intracellular Cleansing as a Natural Healing Method 11
   FINDINGS AND BENEFITS OF INTRACELLULAR CLEANSING 12

CHAPTER 2: DR. SEBI'S ALKALINE DIET 13
   WHAT IS THE ALKALINE DIET? 13
   HOW pH AFFECTS HEALTH (ALKALINE FOODS VS ACIDIC FOODS) 14
   BENEFITS OF THE ALKALINE DIET 14
   LIST OF DR. SEBI APPROVED ALKALINE FOODS 16
   FOODS TO AVOID AT ALL COSTS 17
   HOW TO SWITCH TO THE ALKALINE DIET WITHOUT DIFFICULTY 19

CHAPTER 3: DR. SEBI'S ANTI-INFLAMMATORY DIET 21
   WHAT CAUSES CHRONIC INFLAMMATION IN THE BODY? 21
   ANTI-INFLAMMATORY DIET VS ACIDIC DIET 22
   LIST OF ANTI-INFLAMMATORY FOODS RECOMMENDED BY DR. SEBI 25
      The best natural remedies to reduce inflammation 28

CHAPTER 4: THE HEALING POWER OF HERBS ACCORDING TO DR. SEBI 30
   Why phytotherapy is essential in natural care 31
   HOW TO CHOOSE, BUY, AND STORE MEDICINAL HERBS 31
   Dr. Sebi's 10 Essential Home Pharmacy Herbs 33

CHAPTER 5: SWITCHING TO THE ALKALINE DIET IN 14 DAYS 39
   HOW TO PHASE OUT ACIDIC FOODS WITHOUT STRESS 40
      Examples of toxic or acidifying foods to be eliminated or drastically reduced 40
   HOW TO DEAL WITH DETOX SYMPTOMS 41
      Primary symptoms of detoxification and how to manage them 42
   WEEKLY ALKALINE MENU FOR BEGINNERS 43
      Easy-to-make alkaline snacks and drinks 43
   THE DAILY ROUTINE FOR A HEALTHY AND ALKALINE LIFE 47

CHAPTER 6: DETOX ACCORDING TO DR. SEBI – PURIFYING THE BODY NATURALLY ... 50
   THE IMPORTANCE OF BODY PURIFICATION 51
   Dr. Sebi's 7-Day Detox Plan – How to Do It Safely 51
   THE ROLE OF DETOX WATER AND HERBAL TEAS 53
   How to prepare and take a purifying herbal tea 54

CHAPTER 7: NATURAL LIFESTYLE 56

- The importance of movement and gentle physical activity 57
- The Role of Sleep in Healing the Body 57
  - How to avoid environmental toxins to protect your health 58
  - Emotional Well-Being and Positive Relationships 58
- 10. Energy Rituals and Practices for Wellness 60

CHAPTER 8: NATURAL REMEDIES FOR COMMON DISEASES 63

- Flu and colds 64
- Joint and Muscle Pain 65
  - Dr. Sebi and the conventional modern lines 66
  - Natural Management of Allergies and Asthma 67
  - Concrete Examples of Healing Through the Alkaline Diet 67
- Insomnia and Stress 68
  - Herbs and Natural Remedies 69

CHAPTER 9: DR SEBI AND DIABETES 72

- Refined sugars and acidity in the body 72
- How Alkaline Nutrition Helps Stabilize Blood Sugar 73
- The best herbs to balance blood sugar levels 75
- Smoothies and alkaline recipes for diabetes 76
  - Exercises and daily habits to improve insulin response 80
- Detox techniques to reduce inflammation of the pancreas 81
  - Recommended and Avoiding Foods 83

CHAPTER 10: DR SEBI AND HYPERTENSION 84

- The Real Cause of High Blood Pressure According to Dr. Sebi 84
- Natural herbs to regulate blood pressure 85
  - The Role of Sodium and Potassium in the Alkaline Diet 89
- Strategies to reduce stress and improve circulation 89
- Foods to avoid at all costs for those suffering from hypertension 90
  - Infusions and herbal teas for a healthy heart 92

CHAPTER 11: AUTOIMMUNE DISEASES 97

- The role of inflammation in autoimmune diseases 98
- The connection between mucus, gut, and autoimmune diseases 98
  - Leaky Gut 99
- Microbiota, Prebiotics and Probiotics 99
  - Natural remedies 99
- Herbs and natural remedies to rebalance the immune system 101
- The Power of Alkaline Fasting in Autoimmune Diseases 105
- Stress Management Techniques to Reduce Autoimmune Crises 106
  - Techniques to reduce stress 107
- Strategies to eliminate toxins from the body 108

CHAPTER 12. DR SEBI AND THYROID DISORDERS 111

- How the alkaline diet can rebalance thyroid function 112
  - Antioxidants and thyroid health 113

Holistic approach in the management of thyroid disorders 113
Physical activity and thyroid 113
ESSENTIAL MINERALS FOR A HEALTHY THYROID 114
THE ROLE OF FUCUS VESICULOSUS AND OTHER ALKALINE HERBS 115
FOODS TO AVOID WITH HYPOTHYROIDISM AND HYPERTHYROIDISM 116
THE LINK BETWEEN STRESS, ADRENALINE, AND THYROID HEALTH 117
Natural remedies to improve metabolism and energy 117

CHAPTER 13: HOW TO BOOST THE IMMUNE SYSTEM 119

BEST IMMUNE-BOOSTING HERBS 120
Infusions and decoctions to strengthen natural defenses. 121
Detox routine for the lymphatic system 124

CHAPTER 14: HERPES, HIV AND VIRAL INFECTIONS 126

EFFECTS OF HYPERACIDITY ON METABOLISM 127
More powerful antiviral and antibacterial herbs, according to Dr. Sebi 129
Natural remedies to accelerate the healing of herpes injuries 132
The Role of Stress and Rest in the Treatment of Viral Infections 134
HOW TO DETOXIFY THE BODY OF TOXINS 135

CHAPTER 15: CLEARING MUCUS AND STRENGTHENING THE IMMUNE SYSTEM 139

WHY MUCUS FUELS DISEASE, ACCORDING TO DR. SEBI 140
Central diseases associated with excess mucus 140
What mucus contains 141
Foods that stimulate mucus production are to be avoided 141
Strategies for supplementing a purifying diet 143

CHAPTER 16: NATURAL REMEDIES FOR THE MOST COMMON INFECTIONS 149

HOME REMEDIES FOR TONSILLITIS AND SORE THROAT 150

CHAPTER 17: ANTIVIRAL TONICS AND PURIFICATION PROTOCOLS 159

CHAPTER 18: NATURAL CARE FOR SKIN AND HAIR 168

HAIR HEALTH 169
NATURAL TREATMENTS FOR ECZEMA AND PSORIASIS 170
Herbal Masks & Lotions Recipes 171

CHAPTER 19: DR. SEBI'S FOOD LIST – APPROVED FOODS 174

DR. SEBI'S OFFICIAL LIST IS FRUITS, VEGETABLES, GRAINS, AND LEGUMES 175
WHAT TO EAT AND WHAT TO AVOID 177
Must-Avoid Items 178
NATURAL FOODS AND HYBRID FOODS: WHY AVOID THEM 179
Shopping at the supermarket 182

CHAPTER 20: DR. SEBI STD CURE – NATURAL CURE FOR SEXUALLY TRANSMITTED DISEASES 183

THE LINK BETWEEN DIET AND SEXUALLY TRANSMITTED DISEASES 184
How to get rid of excess mucus 188
NATURAL STRATEGIES TO ELIMINATE EXCESS MUCUS 189

Strengthening the Immune System.. *190*

CHAPTER 21: DR. SEBI DETOX CLEANSE SMOOTHIES – SMOOTHIES FOR DEEP CLEANSING 191

THE IMPORTANCE OF DETOX SMOOTHIES 191
SMOOTHIE RECIPES TO DETOXIFY THE LIVER, INTESTINES, AND BLOOD 192

CHAPTER 22: DR. SEBI HERB'S ENCYCLOPEDIA – THE ENCYCLOPEDIA OF HEALING HERBS 201

THE HERBS OF HONDURAS 202
THE MOST POWERFUL ALKALINE HERBS AND THEIR BENEFITS 203
Key health benefits.. *204*
HOW TO CHOOSE AND USE HERBS FOR SPECIFIC TREATMENTS 206
Phytotherapy and prevention *207*
Drying Techniques... *208*
Conservation Techniques *209*
COMPLETE GUIDE TO PHYTOTHERAPY ACCORDING TO DR. SEBI... 209
Combination of Detox Herbs and Functional Foods *211*
Herb Rotation Strategies... *212*
Contraindications *212*

CONCLUSIONS 213

Don't Miss This!

The Self-Healing Bonus Bundle You'll Wish You Had Sooner...

Hey there,

To thank you for grabbing this book, I've prepared an **exclusive bonus pack** you can download instantly.

Inside, you'll find **practical tools** designed to make your healing journey even easier, more powerful, and more effective—starting *today*.

- **Dr. Sebi's Anti-Mucus Protocol – 5-Day Reset**
- **Printable Daily Tracker for Alkaline Living**
- **Morning Detox & Immunity Rituals Checklist**
- **Top 15 Alkaline Herbs and Their Uses – Mini Cheat Sheet**

These are *not* in the book. They're fast, printable, and perfect for staying on track every day.

Scan the QR code below to access everything for free.

You're going to love this. And honestly? You'd be missing out if you skipped it.
Your body will thank you.

With love,
Emily

INTRODUCTION

Dr. Sebi, whose real name was Alfred Bowman, was born in Honduras and stood out in the natural health landscape thanks to a revolutionary approach. Although he had no formal education, he devoted himself passionately to the self-taught study of the healing properties of plants, developing a method based on the alkaline diet and the use of medicinal herbs.

According to his philosophy, the well-being of the body depended on maintaining a slightly alkaline internal environment capable of counteracting the accumulation of toxins and mucus, which he believed to be responsible for many diseases. This concept of "intracellular cleansing" became the cornerstone of his teaching and attracted the attention of thousands of followers, including numerous celebrities who recognized its effectiveness.

Dr. Sebi's ideas, however, did not fail to arouse controversy: his alternative method led him to clash with official institutions and face legal battles, which, while highlighting the critical side of his statements, helped to consolidate his impact in the field of natural medicine.

Today, Dr. Sebi's legacy inspires those seeking a holistic and conscious approach to well-being, inviting everyone to rediscover the wisdom of nature to live in harmony with their bodies.

Dr. Sebi's method continues to exert a strong impact because it offers a holistic and natural approach to health that resonates with many today. Its emphasis on alkaline dieting, eliminating processed foods, and using medicinal herbs stimulates the body to reconnect with its self-healing abilities, in line with a growing awareness towards healthier, more sustainable lifestyles. In addition, the simplicity and clarity of its principles offer accessible guidance to those looking for alternatives to conventional medicine, making its method a reference point for those who want to take care of their well-being naturally.

To get the maximum benefit from this book, we invite you to read it carefully and actively participate. Take the time to explore each section, following the index that guides you through the fundamental concepts of alkaline diet and herbal medicine, as well as natural remedies and daily routines to improve your well-being. Read each chapter as a practical path: take notes, highlight key tips, and experiment with the proposed recipes and checklists. In this way, you will not only gain in-depth knowledge, but you will be able to turn every suggestion into concrete action, integrating it into your daily life to achieve real and lasting results.

PART 1: DR. SEBI, THE ALKALINE DIET AND PHYTOTHERAPY

CHAPTER 1: WHO WAS DR. SEBI?

Dr. Sebi, born Alfred Bowman, was an herbal healer who revolutionized the concept of natural health. He promoted an alkaline diet and the use of herbs to cleanse the body and restore natural balance. His philosophy is based on the belief that diseases are the result of an accumulation of mucus and toxins in the body caused by an unnatural diet and a lifestyle that is not in harmony with nature.

Dr. Sebi's mission in natural medicine was to rid the body of impurities through an exclusively plant-based diet and the consumption of healing herbs. He firmly believed that the human body was designed to function best with natural, unprocessed foods rich in essential minerals, such as iron, magnesium, and calcium. His approach to healing centered on intracellular cleansing. This concept suggests that health depends on eliminating toxins accumulated over time. Despite not having a traditional medical background, Dr. Sebi gained a global following due to his ability to help people improve their health. However, his method was often challenged by the scientific community and health institutions, leading him to legal battles to defend the validity of his approach. During a historic trial, he presented evidence and testimonies of patients who had been cured thanks to his method, obtaining a sort of legal validation.

Dr. Sebi's message, advocating for a return to a more natural lifestyle free from processed foods and synthetic drugs, continues to inspire many today. His philosophy, centered on the idea that our body possesses an incredible ability to heal itself when provided with the right tools-pure nutrition, adequate hydration, and phytotherapeutic support-aligns with ancient traditions of natural medicine. These traditions, including those of Hippocrates and other holistic healers, also emphasize the crucial role of prevention and balance between body, mind, and spirit, further validating Dr. Sebi's approach.

The concept of intracellular cleaning

Intracellular cleansing is one of the fundamental principles of Dr. Sebi's philosophy. This concept goes beyond simple detoxification and aims to optimize the functioning of cells by eliminating toxins and the balance of body pH. According to this approach, the accumulation of mucus and waste substances inside cells hinders the proper functioning of the body. It is also a determining factor in the development of many chronic diseases.

Dr. Sebi argued that consuming unnatural, acidifying foods (such as processed foods, dairy, meat, and refined sugars) altered the body's normal balance, producing excessive mucus. Instead of being excreted naturally, this mucus accumulates in tissues and organs, hindering the absorption of nutrients and the proper disposal of toxins. When cells are weighed down by waste and impurities, their ability to regenerate and function optimally is impaired, paving the way for chronic inflammation, metabolic imbalances, and even degenerative diseases.

The Role of Mucus and the Link to Disease

Mucus is a substance naturally produced by the body to protect and lubricate tissues, particularly in the respiratory and digestive systems. However, according to Dr. Sebi, excessive mucus production becomes problematic when it accumulates in excess, becoming a breeding ground for bacteria, viruses, and other pathogens.

Scientific studies have highlighted the role of mucus in inflammation and disease. Research published in Frontiers in Immunology suggests that excess pathological mucus can contribute to respiratory disorders such as asthma and chronic obstructive pulmonary disease (COPD) and is associated with digestive disorders such as Crohn's disease and ulcerative colitis. In addition, a Harvard Medical School article explored the link between excess mucus and the increased risk of chronic infections, pointing out how an acidic environment can promote the proliferation of harmful microorganisms.

According to Dr. Sebi's vision, the most common diseases can be classified according to the area of the body where mucus accumulation occurs:

- **The lungs** → can lead to bronchitis, asthma, and pneumonia.
- **In the gut** → can contribute to constipation, irritable bowel, and other digestive diseases.
- **The blood and arteries** → can promote hypertension, circulatory problems, and cardiovascular disorders.
- **The nervous system** → can affect brain function, contributing to cognitive issues, mental fatigue, and brain fog.

Although controversial, this theory is confirmed by studies on the relationship between chronic inflammation and degenerative diseases. For example, research published in Nature Reviews Immunology has shown that systemic inflammation, often triggered by an imbalanced gut microbiota, can negatively affect several organs, from the brain to the heart.

Intracellular Cleansing as a Natural Healing Method

To counteract the accumulation of mucus and toxins, Dr. Sebi proposed a method based on two fundamental pillars:

1. An alkaline diet: A diet based on naturally alkaline foods (such as fruits, green leafy vegetables, seeds, and non-hybridized grains) allows you to restore an optimal pH in the body. Dr. Sebi emphasized that the human body functions best in a slightly alkaline environment (with a pH of around 7.4). In contrast, an acidic environment promotes inflammation and the proliferation of diseases. Numerous studies confirm that a diet rich in plants can reduce chronic inflammation and improve the function of the immune system. For example, research from the University of California has shown that consuming alkaline foods can improve kidney health and reduce the risk of chronic disease.
2. The use of medicinal herbs: Herbal medicine plays a key role in intracellular cleansing, helping the body to eliminate excess mucus and purify the excretory organs (liver, kidneys, intestines, lungs, and skin). Dr. Sebi recommended the use of specific herbs with detox properties, such as:

- Burdock → purifies the blood and supports the liver.
- Sarsaparilla → helps eliminate toxins and improves skin health.
- Nettle → supports kidney function and reduces inflammation.
- Dandelion → stimulates digestion and promotes diuresis.
- Cascara Sagrada → a powerful natural laxative that helps keep your bowels clean.

Studies on Phytotherapy support the use of these plants. For example, research published in Phytotherapy confirmed that burdock has beneficial liver and cell detoxification effects. At the same time, sarsaparilla is known for its purifying action on the blood and its anti-inflammatory properties.

Findings and Benefits of Intracellular Cleansing

Many individuals who have followed Dr. Sebi's method have reported significant benefits, including:

- Increased energy and vitality
- Reduction of joint pain and inflammation
- Improved digestion and intestinal transit
- Better breathing and reduction of nasal and lung congestion
- Healthier, brighter skin by eliminating toxins

These results are consistent with the scientific literature highlighting how an anti-inflammatory diet and herbal remedies can improve human health. For example, an analysis published in The Journal of Nutrition showed that a diet rich in fruits and vegetables reduces the risk of cardiovascular disease and improves immune function. Intracellular cleansing is not just a theoretical concept but a practice that can transform health profoundly. Dr. Sebi has promoted a return to nature, encouraging people to rediscover the body's regenerative power through mindful eating and the use of natural remedies.

Although mainstream medicine does not universally accept his approach, the increasing research focus on alkaline diets, herbal medicine, and detoxification strategies suggests that some aspects of his method merit further exploration. Adopting a lifestyle based on whole foods, pure water, healing herbs, and a balanced body pH can effectively improve overall well-being and prevent many chronic diseases.

CHAPTER 2: DR. SEBI'S ALKALINE DIET

In this chapter, we will delve into the heart of the method proposed by Dr. Sebi, namely the alkaline diet. This dietary approach aims to restore the pH balance in our body and promote health naturally and sustainably. The alkaline diet is not simply a trend of the moment. Still, it represents an authentic lifestyle based on the principle that the body, if properly fed, has intrinsic self-healing abilities. With careful food selection, it is possible to create an internal environment conducive to cell regeneration, reducing the accumulation of toxins and helping to prevent and treat numerous diseases. This chapter is structured to give you a complete overview: from the definition of what an alkaline diet is, through the importance of pH in health, to the practical list of approved foods and foods to avoid, with valuable tips for integrating this dietary philosophy into your daily life.

What is the alkaline diet?

The alkaline diet focuses on eating foods that can keep the body's pH slightly alkaline, typically around neutral or slightly higher. The idea behind this method is that the internal environment of our body, if less acidic, favors the optimal functioning of each cell, improving the ability to regenerate and self-heal. In other words, a favorable acid-base balance helps create the ideal conditions for enzymes and biochemical reactions to operate efficiently, thus reducing the risk of developing chronic diseases.

The basic principle of the alkaline diet is based on the observation that many processed and processed foods – as well as some foods of animal origin – tend to increase acidity in the body. Excess acidity, or systemic acidity, can cause an overload of toxins and inflammation, factors that, according to proponents of this diet, are at the root of numerous disorders and diseases. In contrast, natural, whole, unprocessed foods, such as fresh fruits, leafy greens, nuts, seeds, and non-hybridized whole grains, not only provide essential nutrients but also help keep the body's pH in a slightly alkaline state, thus promoting better cellular health.

This approach is also based on the theory that the human body has natural detoxification mechanisms capable of gradually eliminating accumulated harmful substances. When these processes are supported by a balanced diet free of acidifying foods, the immune system can work more efficiently, improving digestion, nutrient absorption, and circulation, all essential for optimal health.

How pH Affects Health (Alkaline Foods vs Acidic Foods)

pH measures the concentration of hydrogen ions in a solution and indicates how acidic or alkaline it is. In the context of health, the body's pH plays a crucial role because it affects the optimal functioning of enzymes, cellular metabolism, and the immune system's ability to defend itself. A balanced indoor environment, in which the pH remains slightly alkaline, promotes essential biochemical reactions. At the same time, excess acidity can compromise these processes.

The foods we consume have a direct impact on the pH of our bodies. Alkaline foods, such as fresh fruits, leafy greens, cucumbers, and some whole grains, contain minerals and nutrients that help maintain a favorable balance for cellular health. These foods support enzyme function and help neutralize toxins, facilitating the body's detoxification and regeneration processes. Conversely, acidic foods — typically represented by meats, dairy, refined sugars, and processed products — can contribute to an overly acidic internal environment, which in the long term has been associated with inflammatory states and an increased risk of developing chronic disease.

An unbalanced pH, with a predominance of acidity, can, interfere with the proper absorption of nutrients, slow down immune function, and promote inflammatory processes that result in pathological conditions such as diabetes, cardiovascular disease, and even some types of cancer. Therefore, maintaining an optimal acid-base balance is essential to prevent disease onset and support the body's natural self-healing process. Thus, adopting a diet rich in alkaline foods effectively promotes lasting health and reduces the risk of cellular and inflammatory dysfunction.

Benefits of the alkaline diet

An alkaline diet is increasingly recognized for its overall well-being and disease prevention benefits. This dietary approach is based on the principle that the body's acid-base balance is crucial in maintaining optimal health. Maintaining a slightly alkaline body environment helps improve digestion and nutrient absorption. It contributes to reducing systemic inflammation, which underlies many chronic diseases.

Our body's pH varies depending on tissues and organs. The blood, for example, maintains a slightly alkaline pH between 7.35 and 7.45, a fundamental range to ensure normal physiological functions. If this balance is disturbed—for example, due to incorrect eating habits, excessive consumption of processed foods, refined sugars, or animal proteins—the body can accumulate acidic metabolic waste. This waste overloads the mechanisms that regulate pH and can promote the onset of various disorders.

According to research published in *The Journal of Environmental and Public Health*, eating a highly acidic diet (high in processed foods, sugars, red meat, and saturated fats) can impair metabolic functions. Over time, this imbalance increases the risk of chronic inflammation, oxidative stress, and bone loss.

Chronic inflammation is a risk factor linked to numerous diseases, including diabetes, cardiovascular disease, rheumatoid arthritis, and some forms of cancer. A study by the *National Center for Biotechnology Information (NCBI)* found that increasing the consumption of alkaline fruits and vegetables can help lower levels of C-reactive protein (CRP), an indicator of inflammation in the blood.

When the internal environment becomes too acidic, the body can be more exposed to the proliferation of pathogenic bacteria and viruses and facilitate the appearance of degenerative conditions. On the contrary, maintaining a balanced and basically alkaline pH supports immune function. It improves the body's response to external agents.

In practical terms, adopting a diet rich in alkalizing foods means focusing on:

- **Leafy greens** (such as spinach, kale, Swiss chard)
- **Fresh fruit** (especially lemons, avocados, berries, apples)
- **Legumes** (chickpeas, lentils, beans) and whole grains (spelled quinoa, millet)
- **Oilseeds** (pumpkin, sunflower, sesame seeds) and dried fruits (almonds, walnuts)

In addition to food choices, adequate hydration, regular physical activity, and stress management (such as meditation or relaxation techniques) also help keep the body in a more alkaline environment. Our body is designed to self-regulate, but it needs the proper support: a predominantly alkaline diet helps reduce the underlying inflammatory state, promotes the purification of toxins, and offers a less hospitable ground for harmful microorganisms.

The body's pH balance directly affects the digestive system's effectiveness. An organism in an acidic state can experience problems such as gastric reflux, acidity, intestinal dysbiosis, and irritable bowel syndrome.

Consuming alkaline foods promotes better functioning of digestive enzymes, facilitating the assimilation of vitamins, minerals, and other essential nutrients. The integration of plant fibers also improves the health of the intestinal flora, contributing to the growth of beneficial probiotic bacteria and strengthening the intestinal barrier.

A body in acid-base balance has stronger immune defenses. Studies have shown that an alkaline diet improves the body's ability to fight viruses, bacteria, and pathogens, reducing the risk of respiratory and gastrointestinal infections. The alkaline diet is also rich in antioxidants, including vitamins C and E, flavonoids, and polyphenols, which counteract oxidative stress and protect cells from damage caused by free radicals.

One of the lesser-known benefits of the alkaline diet is bone and muscle health. Studies published in the *American Journal of Clinical Nutrition* have shown that excess acidity in the body can lead to the loss of calcium and other essential minerals from the bones, thus increasing the risk of osteoporosis and bone fragility.

To counteract this phenomenon, it is essential to include foods rich in magnesium and potassium, such as spinach, bananas, and almonds, in your diet. These foods help balance the body's pH and improve bone density, reducing the risk of fractures and supporting muscle health.

In addition, a further study published in *Circulation Research* showed that a diet rich in fruits and vegetables, typically alkaline, helps reduce the risk of hypertension and cardiovascular disease. This beneficial effect is due to the ability of alkaline foods to promote the dilation of blood vessels and reduce arterial stiffness, thus contributing to better circulation.

Maintaining a less acidic indoor environment also positively impacts atherosclerotic plaque prevention. High levels of acidity in the blood can damage the walls of the vessels, facilitating the accumulation of LDL cholesterol, the so-called "bad cholesterol." A less acidic body, thanks to a diet rich in alkalizing foods, is therefore less susceptible to this process, helping to protect cardiovascular health in the long term.

Despite its many benefits, the scientific community debates the alkaline diet. Some experts point out that the body already has mechanisms for self-regulating pH, mainly through the kidneys and lungs. That diet only partially affects this balance.

However, clinical studies confirm that a diet rich in alkaline foods and low in processed foods brings tangible benefits, reducing inflammation, improving metabolic health, and promoting overall well-being.

A diet based on alkaline foods can offer extraordinary long-term health benefits by improving acid-base balance, reducing inflammation, and strengthening the body's natural defenses.

Adopting this food philosophy does not mean adhering to rigid rules but rather making more conscious choices that support the well-being of the body. With a more natural diet rich in essential micronutrients, we can prevent many diseases, optimize our vital energy, and promote healthy and harmonious aging.

List of Dr. Sebi Approved Alkaline Foods

Dr. Sebi has identified several foods essential for maintaining the body's alkaline balance, which form the basis of a diet aimed at detoxification and general well-being. These foods are chosen for their nourishing and purifying properties, which can help the body counteract the accumulation of toxins and maintain an optimal pH. Its list includes several categories:

- **Fruits:** Fruits such as apples, pears, grapes, and citrus fruits not only provide vitamins, minerals, and antioxidants but also help to refresh and alkalize the body. Although citrus fruits are acidic by nature, they have an alkalizing effect after digestion.
- **Leafy greens:** Spinach, kale, and lettuce are rich in chlorophyll, vitamins, and minerals that promote detoxification and cell regeneration. These vegetables are among the best allies for counteracting acidity and stimulating the immune system.
- **Other crunchy vegetables:** Cucumbers, peppers, and similar vegetables are known for their high water and mineral content. These foods help to hydrate and cleanse the body, helping to maintain a clean and alkaline indoor environment.
- **Non-hybridized whole grains** and **legumes** provide sustainable energy and nutrients without introducing acidifying substances. Whole grains keep their nutritional properties intact. At the same time, legumes are a valuable source of plant-based protein and fiber.
- **Natural herbs and spices**: Herbs and spices, such as rosemary, thyme, and other medicinal plants, play an essential role in supporting the liver and kidney cleansing processes and possess anti-inflammatory and antioxidant properties.

When consumed regularly, these foods create a solid foundation for an alkaline diet, helping to keep the body in a state conducive to health, cell regeneration, and the prevention of chronic diseases.

Below is a summary table that illustrates some of these foods and their main remedy:

Food	Main Remedy/Benefit
Apples, Pears, Grapes, Citrus Fruits	Provision of vitamins, antioxidants and alkalizing effect after digestion.
Spinach, Kale, Lettuce	Rich in chlorophyll and minerals, they promote purification and cell regeneration.
Cucumbers, Peppers and Crunchy Vegetables	High water and mineral content, they support the body's hydration and purification.
Non-hybridized whole grains	They provide sustainable energy and nutrients without acidifying the body.
Legumes	Source of vegetable protein and fiber, they help maintain a metabolic balance.
Natural Herbs and Spices	Anti-inflammatory, antioxidant properties and support for liver and kidney detoxification.

This selection of foods, when integrated into a daily routine, can contribute significantly to prevention and health improvement, offering a natural and holistic approach that is the basis of Dr. Sebi's method.

Foods to avoid at all costs

To get the maximum benefits from the alkaline diet, it is crucial not only to choose foods that promote a favorable internal environment but also to avoid or drastically reduce those that, on the contrary, tend to acidify the body. The elimination of acidifying foods prevents the accumulation of toxins. It promotes an optimal environment for natural detoxification and self-healing processes. Foods that should be avoided mainly include red meat, dairy products, refined sugars, and processed foods. For various reasons, these products represent a real obstacle to maintaining a healthy acid-base balance.

Red meats, for example, are often high in saturated fats and, during digestion, can contribute to an increase in the body's acidity. Dairy products, despite being a source of protein and calcium, can have an acidifying effect for many individuals, especially if consumed in excess. Refined sugars and processed foods, on the other hand, contain additives and preservatives and lack essential nutrients, causing glycemic spikes and contributing to chronic inflammation, factors that increase the body's acidity.

Reducing or eliminating these foods allows one to avoid overloading with substances that can compromise proper cellular functioning and inhibit self-healing mechanisms. This helps maintain a balanced pH, reduces the risk of developing chronic diseases, and improves digestion, nutrient absorption, and overall energy.

Below is a summary table that explains why it is good to avoid these foods:

Food Category	Motivation to Avoid
Red Meat	Rich in saturated fats and acidifying compounds; They can increase internal acidity and promote inflammation, hindering natural detoxification processes.
Dairy Products	Although they are a source of calcium and protein, they are often acidifying if consumed in excess; they can contribute to pH imbalances, especially in sensitive individuals.
Refined Sugars	Deprived of nutrients and rich in empty calories; They cause glycemic spikes, inflammation and the accumulation of toxins, promoting an acidified internal environment.
Processed Foods	They contain additives, preservatives, and chemicals that alter the body's pH; They lack essential nutrients and can compromise long-term health.

Eliminating these foods or significantly reducing their consumption helps create ideal conditions for the body, allowing cells to function at their best and fully take advantage of the body's regenerative power. This dietary change is not just a style choice but a real investment in one's health and well-being, in line with the philosophy of the alkaline diet.

A thought on saturated fats

Saturated fats are a type of fat in which the fatty acid chains do not have double bonds, which makes them solid at room temperature. Excessive consumption of these fats can harm the body because it increases the level of bad cholesterol (LDL) in the blood. This can lead to plaque forming in the arteries, making them stiffer and increasing the risk of cardiovascular problems, such as heart attack and stroke. In addition, too much-saturated fat can promote inflammatory processes and disrupt normal metabolism, contributing to other health problems.

Vegetable fibers

Dietary fiber plays a vital role in the overall health and well-being of the body. First, fiber helps maintain a healthy body weight. Slowing digestion and prolonging the sense of satiety prevents overeating and sudden hunger peaks. This effect is because fiber, especially soluble fiber, forms a kind of gel in the stomach that slows down the absorption of nutrients, stabilizing blood sugar levels and contributing to a longer-lasting feeling of fullness. In addition, insoluble fibers act directly on intestinal transit, promoting regularity and preventing constipation while helping to prevent the formation of problems such as hemorrhoids or diverticulitis.

Fiber plays a key role in cleansing the intestine. Stimulating stool transit facilitates the natural elimination of toxins and residues accumulated in the digestive tract, thus helping to maintain a healthy intestinal environment and reduce the risk of chronic inflammation. A well-functioning intestine also promotes a balance of bacterial flora, a crucial element for an efficient immune system and general well-being.

This is especially important when considering the dietary approach proposed by Dr. Sebi, who advocated the importance of a diet based on natural, whole foods. His philosophy aimed to create a less acidic and more balanced internal environment where nutrient-rich foods – such as fruits, vegetables, whole grains, legumes, and nuts – play a key role. In addition to supporting digestive health, fiber helps maintain an efficient metabolism and prevent the accumulation of toxins, essential elements to support the body's natural self-healing process. Regular dietary fiber intake helps improve the immune response, as a clean and well-balanced gut promotes better assimilation of nutrients and reduces systemic inflammatory load. This synergy between foods rich in fiber and other nutrients promotes better circulation and a general biochemical balance of the body, which Dr. Sebi considers essential to maintain optimal health and prevent numerous diseases.

The diet proposed by Dr. Sebi, based on whole and natural foods, encourages a holistic approach to well-being. Fiber consumption becomes an essential tool to improve intestinal function and promote greater mental clarity, constant energy, and a better quality of life. Adopting this type of diet means investing in health daily, creating the ideal conditions for a body to be in balance and heal itself over time.

How to switch to the alkaline diet without difficulty

Switching to an alkaline diet does not mean radically upsetting your lifestyle overnight but instead making a series of small, gradual changes that, over time, translate into concrete health benefits. Suppose you're tired of feeling overwhelmed by crash diets and looking for a sustainable approach that fits your daily routine. In that case, this path is designed just for you. Imagine transforming, day after day, eating habits with simple substitutions that allow you to enjoy more natural and purifying foods without sudden sacrifices or extreme sacrifices.

The first step is to know well which foods are acidifying and which, on the other hand, promote an alkaline environment. You could start by gradually replacing foods that currently make your body more acidic — such as red meats, dairy, refined sugars, and processed foods — with alternatives that support pH balance, such as opting for fresh fruits, leafy greens, and non-hybridized whole grains. Planning balanced weekly menus and experimenting with simple recipes based on these ingredients can be a great way to familiarize yourself with your new diet, making the transition less intimidating and more fun.

Using practical tools, such as checklists and daily routines, will help you track your progress and goals. For example, you could start each morning with a glass of warm lemon water to stimulate your detoxification system or schedule a post-lunch walk to aid digestion and reduce stress, which can affect your body's pH. The goal is to create a series of positive habits that, accumulated over time, will make the transition to the alkaline diet fluid and natural without the sense of deprivation or discomfort of diets that are too rigid.

Below is a simple list of practical tips to facilitate this step:

1. **Start with small changes:** You don't need to revolutionize your diet overnight. You can start by gradually replacing some acidifying foods — such as processed meats and refined sugars — with more alkaline options, such as fresh fruits and vegetables. This step-by-step approach allows your body to adapt without feeling overwhelmed.
2. **Plan weekly menus:** Plan meals weekly by creating simple and balanced recipes. Focus on dishes made with fruits, vegetables, whole grains, and legumes, which provide essential nutrients and help keep the pH balanced. Planning enables you to avoid impulsive choices and ensure variety in your diet.
3. **Use daily checklists and routines:** Keep track of your meals and habits with a checklist or food diary. This allows you to track progress, identify any areas for improvement, and stay motivated to eat a more balanced and natural diet.
4. **Hydration in the morning:** Start your day by drinking warm water with a squeeze of lemon. This simple ritual helps stimulate the digestive system, promotes detoxification, and prepares the body to absorb nutrients from subsequent meals better.
5. **Pay attention to portions:** Eating slowly and mindfully is essential to recognize the signs of satiety. Take the time to enjoy each bite. This not only improves digestion but also avoids overeating, helping to maintain a healthy weight.
6. **Integrate light physical activity:** After meals, a short walk or light physical activity can stimulate digestion and reduce stress. Exercise also helps maintain an active metabolism and improve mood, completing the picture of a healthy lifestyle.
7. **Experiment and learn:** Don't be afraid to try new recipes and find out which alkaline foods you like best. The cooking experience can make the transition to a more natural diet more enjoyable and allow you to customize your diet to your preferences and needs.

Taking these simple steps will allow you to integrate the alkaline diet into your life gradually and sustainably, improving your overall well-being without stress and in a concrete way.

CHAPTER 3: DR. SEBI'S ANTI-INFLAMMATORY DIET

The anti-inflammatory diet is one of the most effective approaches to counteract the silent disease that creeps into our body daily: chronic inflammation. Although initially a natural defense reaction of the body against external aggressions such as infections, trauma, or toxins, this process can, if prolonged over time, become a sneaky enemy that compromises general well-being. Chronic inflammation is, in fact, the basis of many diseases, from joint irritations to systemic diseases such as diabetes, cardiovascular diseases, and even some forms of cancer.

Throughout this chapter, we will explore in depth the link between diet and inflammation, analyzing how a well-structured diet can positively influence the level of inflammation in the body. We will start with an overview of the factors that trigger chronic inflammation, focusing on the mechanisms that favor the accumulation of toxins and the development of harmful inflammatory states in the presence of an acid-base imbalance.

Next, we will compare two opposing dietary approaches: on the one hand, the anti-inflammatory diet, rich in natural and nutritious foods that help maintain a balanced internal environment conducive to cell regeneration; on the other, the acidic diet, characterized by processed foods, refined sugars, red meat, and other foods that tend to trigger and perpetuate inflammatory states. We will analyze how this imbalance can lead to a deterioration of the immune system, negatively affect digestion, and trigger inflammatory chain reactions that, in the long term, put the health of the body at risk.

Dr. Sebi's philosophy offers concrete and practical insights in this context. Adopting an anti-inflammatory diet based on the intake of foods that promote pH balance and the elimination of toxins is possible not only to prevent the onset of diseases but also to reverse the cellular and metabolic damage accumulated over time. The benefits of this approach extend beyond simply reducing inflammation: a diet rich in cleansing foods promotes digestion, improves nutrient absorption, stimulates the immune system, and, in general, increases the level of energy and vitality, making the body more resilient to daily aggressions.

What causes chronic inflammation in the body?

Chronic inflammation in the body is not the result of a single isolated factor but of a combination of elements that, interacting with each other, trigger a prolonged and often silent inflammatory response. A key aspect is an unbalanced lifestyle, characterized by a lack of regular physical activity, insufficient sleep, and high-stress levels. Stress induces the release of hormones such as cortisol, which, if produced in excess and for prolonged periods, can alter the normal immune balance and promote a constant inflammatory state.

In addition to stress, daily exposure to toxic substances in the environment—such as air pollutants, pesticides, and chemicals found in industrial products—contributes to increasing the toxic load on our bodies. Once accumulated, these toxins can interfere with normal cellular functioning, causing damage and inflammation at a microscopic level.

Another key element is incorrect nutrition. Excessive consumption of highly processed foods, refined sugars, saturated fats, and acidifying foods contributes to an excessively acidic internal environment. This imbalance in body pH, combined with the lack of essential nutrients and antioxidants, promotes the accumulation of toxins and the onset of inflammatory processes. The body, unable to adequately eliminate these harmful substances, begins to respond with constant inflammation, which, over time, can compromise cellular balance and predispose to the development of chronic diseases such as diabetes, cardiovascular disease, and other degenerative conditions.

Finally, chronic inflammation can also be fueled by psychological and environmental factors that weaken the body's natural defenses. The combination of a stressful lifestyle, exposure to toxins, and poor nutrition creates a vicious circle: the accumulation of toxins and acidifying substances causes persistent inflammation, which in turn interferes with the body's regular self-healing and cleansing process, further aggravating the long-term state of health.

Anti-inflammatory diet vs acidic diet

The anti-inflammatory and acidic diets represent two opposite approaches that profoundly affect the functioning of our body. On the one hand, the anti-inflammatory diet focuses on the intake of foods that promote a balanced internal environment that is less susceptible to inflammation. These foods, rich in nutrients, vitamins, minerals, and antioxidants, help neutralize free radicals and reduce inflammatory processes, allowing cells to repair and regenerate more effectively. An anti-inflammatory diet based on fruits, vegetables, legumes, whole grains, and medicinal herbs supports normal digestive and immune processes. It helps keep the body's pH slightly alkaline, a condition favorable to cellular health.

On the other hand, the acidic diet is characterized by the predominant consumption of foods that tend to generate a more acidic internal environment, such as red meat, dairy products, processed foods, refined sugars, and many industrial drinks. These foods, often poor in essential nutrients, fail to support self-healing processes and can trigger inflammatory reactions that, over time, contribute to the onset of chronic diseases. Excess acidity in the body can alter the proper functioning of enzymes, interfere with digestion, and weaken the immune system, creating a breeding ground for systemic inflammation and metabolic disorders.

The comparison between these two approaches highlights how consuming acidifying foods can lead to chronic inflammation, compromising the efficiency of the body's repair processes. On the other hand, a diet based on natural and alkalizing foods, typical of the anti-inflammatory approach, reduces the risk of inflammation and supports the body's ability to eliminate toxins and maintain an optimal balance. This promotes cell regeneration, the efficient functioning of the immune system, and better management of oxidative stress.

While an acidic diet can trigger and perpetuate harmful inflammatory processes, adopting an anti-inflammatory diet offers an effective path to restoring internal harmony and promoting long-lasting health. This contrast highlights the importance of making conscious food choices oriented towards foods that not only nourish the body but also help it protect and regenerate naturally.

Acidic foods and scientific studies

In recent decades, the adoption of particularly restrictive or extreme diets has gained more and more attention, so much so that some have proclaimed it as the key to health and the prevention of many diseases. However, a significant part of the scientific community has warned of the adverse effects that such approaches can have in the long run. Several studies have shown that, although a well-planned and targeted diet can bring clear benefits in weight control and improved quality of life, the prolonged adoption of excessively restrictive diets can carry considerable risks.

The main problem lies in the possibility of developing nutritional deficiencies since the elimination or extreme limitation of certain foods can deprive the body of vitamins, minerals, and other essential nutrients. In addition, scientific studies have highlighted how the body, in response to prolonged calorie restrictions, can adapt by reducing the basal metabolic rate, negatively impacting long-term weight maintenance. Not only that, but some data also suggest that such diets can negatively affect cardiovascular health and even cognitive function, contributing to the development of mood disorders and alterations in mental well-being.

The literature also raises the issue of effects on intestinal function: the lack of a food variety can alter the balance of bacterial flora, compromising digestion and the immune system. Given these potential risks, it is crucial to carefully analyze the scientific evidence and understand that nutritional balance is essential for maintaining long-term health.

Below are listed the main studies and scientific evidence that highlight the negative effects of prolonged and overly restrictive diets, emphasizing the importance of a balanced and sustainable approach to nutrition.

Risk of nutritional deficiencies

A diet that is too restrictive can significantly reduce the intake of essential vitamins and minerals. These substances, including vitamin D, calcium, iron, and essential fatty acids, are necessary for ensuring the correct functioning of the body. Their deficiency can weaken the immune system, increase susceptibility to infections and diseases, compromise bone health, and predispose to conditions such as osteopenia or osteoporosis. Furthermore, according to some publications in the Journal of the American Medical Association (JAMA), when you eliminate entire food groups, you become more likely to incur nutritional imbalances that, if neglected, can lead to chronic and difficult-to-correct problems.

For health-conscious people, it is essential to remember that not all nutrients can be easily replaced with supplements. Often, a natural and balanced diet remains the best way to obtain a complete intake of micronutrients. If supplementary support is necessary, it is always advisable to contact a nutrition professional.

Metabolic imbalances and slow metabolism

One of the most common adaptations when following an excessively low-calorie or restrictive diet is slowing the basal metabolism. The body, perceiving a "famine," tries to conserve as much energy as possible, lowering caloric expenditure and reducing the ability to burn fat. Studies conducted by various research centers have highlighted how this prolonged reaction can make it challenging to maintain a healthy weight and increase the risk of regaining the lost pounds with interest (the "yo-yo" effect). For those who want long-lasting results, the key lies in moderation and gradualness. A slight calorie deficit, combined with adequate physical training and a good balance of macronutrients (proteins, carbohydrates, and fats), helps prevent the body's "defense" reactions and promotes sustainable weight loss over time.

Impact on cardiovascular health

A diet that is too strict can compromise heart health. According to some studies published in The Lancet, a strong reduction in nutrients and the increase in oxidative stress linked to an unbalanced diet can contribute to alterations in cardiovascular function. In the long term, this could translate into a greater risk of developing diseases such as hypertension, arteriosclerosis, or other heart problems.

For those who practice sports or are particularly active, a balanced diet rich in antioxidants (fruit and vegetables), good fatty acids (for example, those contained in oily fish and dried fruit), and complex carbohydrates help protect the heart and support physical performance. Drastically reducing some macronutrients or following "monothematic" diets (based on a single food or group of foods) can weaken the cardiovascular system.

Effects on cognitive function and mood

Highly restrictive diets can also have significant repercussions on mental well-being. Some research in the nutritional and psychological fields has highlighted how a reduced intake of energy and essential nutrients can favor the onset of mood disorders, including depression and anxiety. Furthermore, alterations in the perception of food and one's body can occur, sometimes paving the way for actual eating disorders. For those who want a holistic approach to well-being, remember that the mind and body are closely interconnected. Following a balanced diet, which includes all macronutrients and a good variety of micronutrients, supports brain function and helps maintain emotional balance, reducing the risk of depressive and anxious states.

Alterations in intestinal function

An aspect that is often underestimated concerns intestinal health. According to the British Journal of Nutrition, eliminating entire categories of foods for long periods can negatively affect the intestinal bacterial flora (microbiota), causing imbalances that can result in digestive problems, abdominal swelling, and alterations in transit. A healthy microbiota is crucial for proper digestion, the functionality of the immune system, and general well-being.

For those looking to improve the quality of daily life, introducing a good variety of foods rich in fiber (whole grains, legumes, fruits, and vegetables) and sources of probiotics (yogurt, kefir, fermented foods) helps maintain the balance of the intestinal flora. Avoiding diets that eliminate one or more food groups is the first step to maintaining the health of the gastrointestinal tract. These studies show that although there are numerous benefits to adopting a healthy and balanced diet, it is essential to avoid restrictions that are too extreme or prolonged over time. Maintaining an adequate nutritional balance, supplementing various foods, and monitoring nutrient intake are vital to preserving overall health in the long run.

List of anti-inflammatory foods recommended by Dr. Sebi

Thanks to their nutritional and antioxidant properties, Dr. Sebi recommended a wide variety of anti-inflammatory foods that help neutralize free radicals and keep the body in balance. These foods, mainly of plant origin, can reduce the toxic load, promote detoxification, and contribute to a more alkaline internal environment, which is essential for limiting inflammatory processes. Regularly incorporating these foods into your diet can support cell regeneration, improve digestion, and strengthen the immune system.

Among the main anti-inflammatory foods recommended by Dr. Sebi are fruits, vegetables, non-hybridized whole grains, legumes, and a selection of medicinal herbs. For example, fresh fruits such as apples, pears, and citrus fruits provide vitamins and minerals and have an alkalizing effect after digestion. Leafy green vegetables, such as spinach and kale, are rich in chlorophyll and nutrients that help cleanse the body and reduce inflammation. In addition, crunchy vegetables such as cucumbers and peppers support the hydration and cleansing of cells due to their high water and mineral content. Whole grains and legumes, chosen in their most natural form, provide fiber and vegetable proteins without weighing down the system with acidifying substances. Finally, natural herbs and spices such as rosemary, thyme, ginger, and turmeric, in addition to having direct anti-inflammatory properties, play a fundamental role in stimulating liver and kidney detoxification processes.

To make it easier to integrate these foods into your daily life, here is a summary table that illustrates some of the anti-inflammatory foods recommended by Dr. Sebi and their main benefit:

Food	Main Benefit
Apples and Pears	Rich in fiber and antioxidants; alkalizing effect post-digestion and immune system support.
Citrus fruits (lemons, oranges)	They provide vitamin C and alkalizing compounds; They help neutralize free radicals and promote purification.
Spinach and Kale	Rich in chlorophyll, vitamins and minerals; They support detoxification and reduce inflammation.
Cucumbers and Peppers	High water and mineral content; they promote hydration and cellular cleansing.
Non-hybridized whole grains	Sustainable energy source and fiber; they help maintain pH balance without acidifying the body.
Legumes	Source of vegetable protein and fiber; They support healthy digestion and reduce inflammation.
Ginger and Turmeric	Known anti-inflammatory and antioxidant properties; They help reduce pain and systemic inflammation.
Rosemary and Thyme	They stimulate detoxification and have anti-inflammatory effects; improve circulation and metabolism.

This list is a good starting point for those who want to follow Dr. Sebi's method and adopt a diet that reduces inflammation naturally. Incorporating these foods into your daily routine can make all the difference in promoting lasting well-being and counteracting the negative effects of a modernly stressful and often over-acidifying lifestyle.

Anti-inflammatory Detox Smoothie (Breakfast or Snack)

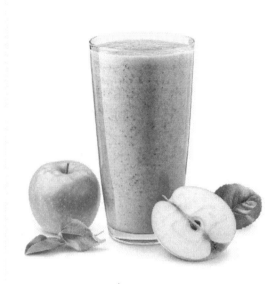

It reduces inflammation, supports digestion and hydration, provides antioxidants.

Ingredients:

- 1 green apple or pear
- 1/2 cucumber
- Juice of 1/2 lemon
- 1 piece of fresh ginger (2 cm)
- 1 handful of spinach
- 1 glass of coconut water or plain water
- 1/2 teaspoon turmeric powder
- 1 teaspoon chia seeds (optional, for extra fiber)

Preparation:

1. Put all the ingredients in the blender and blend until smooth.
2. Drink immediately to maximize the nutritional benefits.

Energizing Hydrating Salad (Lunch)

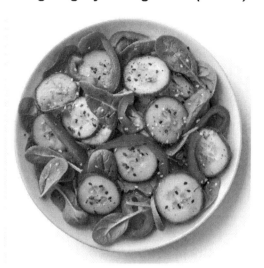

It improves cellular hydration, provides fiber and minerals, helps detoxification.

Ingredients:

- 1 cucumber
- 1 red pepper
- 1 handful of spinach or kale
- 1/2 avocado
- Juice of 1/2 lemon
- 1 tablespoon of extra virgin olive oil
- 1 pinch of pink Himalayan salt
- 1 sprig of fresh thyme

Preparation:

1. Cut the cucumber and bell pepper into thin slices.
2. Combine the vegetables with the spinach or kale in a bowl.
3. Add the diced avocado and season with lemon juice, olive oil, and fresh thyme.
4. Mix well and serve immediately.

Creamy Legume and Turmeric Soup (Dinner)

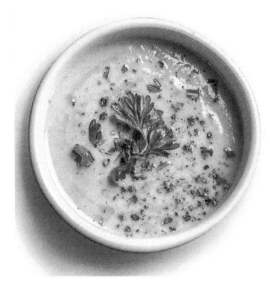

It supports the immune system, promotes digestion, reduces inflammation and provides plant protein.

Ingredients:

- 1 cup of mixed legumes (chickpeas, beans) already cooked
- 1 carrot
- 1 stalk of celery
- 1/2 onion
- 1 clove of garlic
- 1/2 teaspoon turmeric powder
- 1 teaspoon chopped fresh rosemary
- 1 teaspoon of extra virgin olive oil
- 3 cups vegetable broth

Preparation:

1. In a pot, sauté onion, garlic, carrot, and celery with olive oil for 5 minutes.
2. Add the cooked legumes, vegetable broth, turmeric and rosemary.
3. Cook for 15 minutes, then blend half of the soup to get a creamy consistency.
4. Serve hot with a drizzle of raw oil.

Quinoa and Apple Porridge with Cinnamon (Breakfast)

It provides sustainable energy, balances pH and improves metabolism.

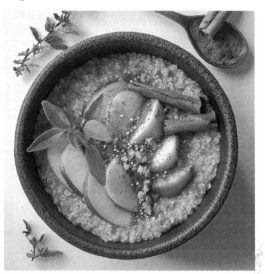

Ingredients:

- 1/2 cup of unhybridized whole wheat quinoa
- 1 apple cut into cubes
- 1 cup sugar-free almond milk
- 1/2 teaspoon ground cinnamon
- 1 teaspoon of honey or agave syrup
- 1 handful of ground almonds

Preparation:

1. Cook the quinoa in almond milk for 10-15 minutes.
2. Add the diced apple and cinnamon, stirring well.
3. Let it cook for another 5 minutes until creamy.
4. Garnish with chopped almonds and a drizzle of honey before serving.

Detox Herbal Tea with Rosemary, Thyme and Lemon (After Dinner or During the Day)

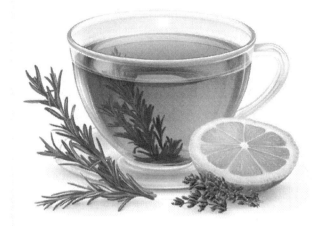

It promotes purification, improves circulation and supports digestion.

Ingredients

- 1 sprig of fresh rosemary
- 1 sprig of fresh thyme
- Juice of 1/2 lemon
- 1 cup of hot water

Preparation

1. Bring the water to a boil and pour over the rosemary and thyme.
2. Leave to infuse for 10 minutes.
3. Add the lemon juice and stir well before drinking.

The best natural remedies to reduce inflammation

In addition to the careful choice of foods, there are numerous natural remedies that, if integrated into a balanced diet, can significantly contribute to reducing inflammation. These remedies not only act directly against inflammatory processes, but also stimulate the body's natural detoxification mechanisms, supporting the immune system and promoting a cleaner and more harmonious internal environment. The use of herbs, herbal teas and complementary practices represents an integrated approach that works on several levels: from the reduction of oxidative stress to the improvement of circulation, to the optimization of cellular metabolism. The combination of these tools allows you to create a holistic strategy to prevent and mitigate the symptoms of chronic conditions, promoting long-lasting health and overall well-being.

These natural remedies include not only taking specific herbal teas and anti-inflammatory herbal infusions, but also practices such as meditation, light physical activity, and breathing techniques that promote calmness and detoxification. These practices act in synergy with a diet rich in alkaline and anti-inflammatory foods, enhancing the overall effect and helping the body to rebalance its internal environment. For example, herbal teas made with ginger, turmeric, or chamomile tea can provide immediate relief from inflammatory symptoms, while regular use of herbs such as rosemary and thyme helps stimulate circulation and facilitate the elimination of accumulated toxins.

Here is a simple list of the best natural remedies to reduce inflammation:

Managing inflammation is a crucial aspect of keeping the body in balance and preventing oxidative stress, muscle stiffness, and other related disorders. Dr. Sebi, among his many teachings, highlighted the importance of integrating natural remedies into one's daily routine which, thanks to their anti-inflammatory properties, help reduce acidity and counteract stress.

- **Ginger:** Infused or added to recipes, it possesses strong anti-inflammatory properties and helps reduce pain and inflammation.
- **Turmeric:** Used in golden milk, herbal teas or supplements, it is recognized for its powerful antioxidant and anti-inflammatory effect.
- **Chamomile:** Chamomile tea calms the nervous system and helps reduce internal inflammation.
- **Rosemary and Thyme:** These aromatic herbs stimulate circulation, support detoxification and have anti-inflammatory properties.
- **Green tea:** Rich in antioxidants, it helps reduce oxidative stress and inflammation.
- **Fennel infusion:** Promotes healthy digestion and reduces inflammation in the intestine.
- **Garlic:** Known for its antibacterial and anti-inflammatory properties, garlic can be integrated into recipes to support the immune system.
- **Bromelain:** An enzyme found in papaya that is known to reduce inflammation and aid digestion.
- **Holy Basil (Tulsi):** This adaptogenic herb helps reduce stress and possesses anti-inflammatory properties.
- **Extra virgin olive oil:** Rich in antioxidants and healthy fats, it supports cardiovascular health and reduces inflammation.
- **Warm lemon water:** Starting your day with this ritual helps stimulate your detoxification system and maintain pH balance.
- **Breathing Techniques and Meditation:** Practices that reduce stress, one of the main triggers of chronic inflammation.
- **Light physical activity:** Daily walks, yoga or stretching improve circulation and promote general well-being.
- **Steam baths:** Useful for opening pores and stimulating the elimination of toxins, helping to reduce inflammation.
- **Lymphatic drainage massages:** They help stimulate the lymphatic system and facilitate the elimination of toxins from the body.

Incorporating these remedies into your daily routine will allow you to support the body's self-healing process and counteract the negative effects of acidity and stress. We recommend that you always have one or more of these remedies on hand, so that you can easily use them in case of need and thus help maintain optimal internal balance and lasting health. By adopting this approach, also inspired by Dr. Sebi's philosophy, you can transform small daily habits into powerful tools for overall well-being.

CHAPTER 4: THE HEALING POWER OF HERBS ACCORDING TO DR. SEBI

The healing power of plants promotes the overall well-being of the body and mind. Since ancient times, civilizations worldwide have recognized and passed down knowledge of medicinal herbs from generation to generation, using them to address health problems, prevent disease, and support healing processes. Over the centuries, these traditions have been enriched by empirical observation and experience, constituting an invaluable heritage of knowledge from which we can still benefit today.

In this chapter, we will dive into the vast and fascinating universe of phytotherapy, exploring how medicinal plants can intervene in a complementary way to a natural diet and other holistic remedies to restore the balance and harmony of the body. Unlike synthetic drugs, which often suppress symptoms, herbs work synergistically with the body's physiological processes, gently supporting and stimulating them. Each plant, in fact, has unique and specific properties that can act on multiple aspects of health, from deep detoxification to anti-inflammatory action, from strengthening the immune system to regulating digestive and metabolic processes.

Ancient wisdom, handed down from generation to generation, teaches us that nature is a real open-air pharmacy. Understanding and respecting each herb's properties allows us to treat the symptoms of malaise and act more deeply, restoring those internal balances often altered by stress, pollution, improper nutrition, and a hectic lifestyle. Therefore, conscious use of medicinal plants can become a valuable ally in preventing numerous diseases and strengthening the body, making it more resilient to external attacks and daily challenges.

Phytotherapy integrates perfectly with the philosophy of a natural and balanced diet. While the diet provides essential nutrients to maintain a good level of energy and health, herbs can act as "specialists" in particular areas, carrying out targeted actions: for example, some plant substances help protect the liver, others support kidney function, others regulate mood or enhance the immune response. This synergy between plants and nutrition makes it possible to create a complete treatment path in which the body is supported at 360 degrees, both in the preventive and recovery phases.

Importantly, herbal medicine masks symptoms and aims to act sincerely, stimulating the body's intrinsic self-healing mechanisms. In addition to being less invasive, this approach respects the body's natural rhythms. It contributes to the construction of solid and lasting health. This is why, in the context of a global method such as that of Dr. Sebi, medicinal herbs become a fundamental element. By integrating the benefits of a natural diet with the healing power that only nature can offer, we can embark on a path toward practical, sustainable health and perfect harmony with our biological rhythm.

Why phytotherapy is essential in natural care

Phytotherapy is a fundamental pillar of natural medicine, as it exploits the healing properties of medicinal plants to harmoniously and gradually restore the body's balance. Unlike synthetic drugs, which often suppress symptoms without resolving the root causes of ailments, plants work synergistically with the body's biological processes, stimulating its innate self-healing abilities. This approach allows you to effectively address health problems and promotes more profound and longer-lasting cell regeneration.

Medicinal herbs have a complex and multifactorial action, thanks to the natural combination of numerous active ingredients that work in perfect synergy. This means that, instead of providing a unidirectional and aggressive effect, as with many pharmacological treatments, phytotherapy acts on different levels, supporting and rebalancing the body's functions. For example, many plants relieve the symptoms of a disorder and intervene in its origins, helping to strengthen the immune system, improve blood circulation, and facilitate detoxification. This makes herbal treatments particularly suitable for treating diseases already in progress and prevention, as they keep the body in an optimal state of well-being and enhance its resilience to external agents.

One of the most valuable aspects of phytotherapy is its ability to promote the rebalancing of the body without overloading it with aggressive chemicals. Many modern ailments result from the accumulation of toxins, chronic inflammation, and oxidative stress, which impair the normal functioning of organs and tissues. Medicinal plants, thanks to their purifying and antioxidant properties, help eliminate impurities, reduce inflammation, and promote a healthier and more alkaline internal environment. This natural cleansing effect is particularly evident in herbs that support the liver, kidneys, and lymphatic system, facilitating the elimination of metabolic waste products and improving the efficiency of the whole body.

An additional benefit of herbal medicine is its compatibility with other holistic approaches, such as a balanced diet, meditation, and relaxation practices. The conscious use of medicinal plants, in fact, is not limited to the simple intake of herbal teas or extracts but can become an integral part of a broader wellness path aimed at restoring harmony between body and mind. This means that, in addition to treating specific ailments, herbal medicine can help improve the quality of life, promoting greater vitality, better emotional balance, and a more remarkable ability to cope with daily stress.

Therefore, the knowledge and use of medicinal herbs represent an invaluable resource for those who want to adopt a more natural and sustainable approach to health. Thanks to their gentle but effective action, plants can accompany the body in a progressive and profound healing process, stimulating its defense mechanisms without altering its balance. In a world increasingly exposed to artificial substances and invasive treatments, rediscovering the therapeutic power of nature means taking a step towards a more conscious, respectful, and lasting health.

How to choose, buy, and store medicinal herbs

When you integrate medicinal herbs into your wellness journey, paying particular attention to several aspects, starting with choosing herbs, is essential. It is necessary to favor those grown organically or spontaneously in unpolluted areas where nature can fully express its healing properties. In addition, it is preferable to opt for herbs harvested when the plant reaches the peak of its therapeutic qualities, as this directly affects the concentration of active ingredients. When buying packaged products, it is advisable to always check the origin and certifications to ensure that you receive an authentic and high-quality product.

Another aspect to consider concerns the part of the plant used. Medicinal plants, in fact, can accumulate active ingredients in different sections, such as leaves, roots, flowers, or seeds, and each can offer specific benefits. For example, ginger root is particularly renowned for its anti-inflammatory properties. At the same time, lavender flowers are prized for the calming and relaxing compounds they contain. Knowing which part of the plant most suits your therapeutic goal allows you to make a more informed and targeted choice.

It is also essential to inquire thoroughly about the therapeutic interest of the herb you intend to use, evaluating the benefits and any contraindications or interactions with other drugs. In this context, the advice of an herbalist or qualified professional can be invaluable in avoiding risks and maximizing the remedy's effectiveness.

Moving on to the time of purchase, it is preferable to contact herbalists or specialized shops, where the staff can provide expert and personalized advice. Buying from improvised retailers or markets where the origin is unclear can involve risks in terms of the quality and authenticity of the product. If you buy online, it is essential to choose specialized e-commerce sites that offer detailed data sheets on the cultivation and processing of herbs, as well as checking reviews and manufacturer transparency. In addition, herbs come in different forms: dried leaves and roots, mother tinctures, capsules, or powders. The choice of the most suitable shape depends on the intended use. For example, dried leaves are ideal for making herbal teas and infusions. At the same time, tinctures or liquid extracts may be more practical for quick and concentrated intake.

Once purchased, it is equally essential to know and correctly apply preservation techniques to preserve the active properties of herbs. In a calm, dry environment, herbs should be placed in airtight containers, preferably glass, and kept away from direct light and moisture. This helps to keep the aroma and beneficial substances intact. It is important to remember that herbs have a limited shelf life: generally, dried leaves retain their properties for about a year, while flowers deteriorate more quickly. For this reason, it is helpful to mark the date of purchase on the jars or packages and check the state of conservation regularly. Suppose you notice any changes in color, an unpleasant odor, or mold. In that case, it is advisable to discard the product so that you always use safe and active herbs.

Dr. Sebi's 10 Essential Home Pharmacy Herbs

Burdock: Known for its detoxifying properties, it helps rid the body of accumulated toxins and supports skin health.

Burdock Detox Infusion (To eliminate toxins and improve skin)

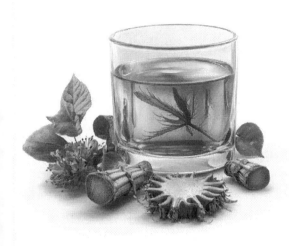

Ingredients:

- 1 tablespoon dried burdock root
- 250 ml of water
- Juice of half a lemon (optional)

Preparation:

1. Bring the water to a boil and add the burdock root.
2. Leave to infuse for 10-15 minutes, then filter.
3. Add lemon juice to enhance the detox effect and drink once a day.

Sarsaparilla Purifying Decoction (To purify the blood)

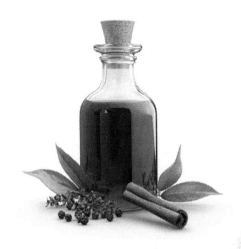

Ingredients:

- 1 tablespoon of sarsaparilla root
- 300 ml of water
- 1 teaspoon of natural honey (optional)

Preparation:

1. Boil the water, add the sarsaparilla root and let it simmer for 20 minutes.
2. Strain and sweeten with honey if desired.
3. Drink lukewarm once a day.

Digestive Herbal Tea with Cascara Sagrada
(To facilitate digestion and intestinal transit)

Known for cleansing the intestines, it facilitates intestinal transit and promotes proper digestion.

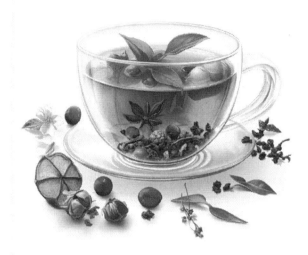

Ingredients:

- 1/2 teaspoon dried cascara sagrada bark
- 250 ml boiling water
- 1 slice of ginger (optional)

Preparation:

1. Pour boiling water over the cascara sagrada.
2. Leave to infuse for 5 minutes (no longer, to avoid excessive laxative effects).
3. Filter and drink before bed, no more than 3 times a week.

Nettle Green Juice *(To support the kidneys and purify the urinary system)*

Acts as kidney support, helping to cleanse the urinary system and eliminate toxins.

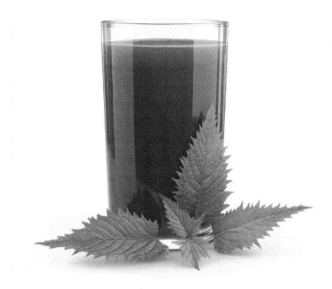

Ingredients:

- 1 handful of fresh nettle leaves (or 1 teaspoon of dried nettle)
- 1 cucumber
- 1 green apple
- Juice of 1/2 lemon
- 250 ml of water

Preparation:

1. Blend all the ingredients until you get a smooth juice.
2. Strain if you prefer a more liquid consistency.
3. Drink cool in the morning to maximize the purifying effect.

Fucus Vesiculosus Mineral Broth (To support thyroid and metabolism)

Rich in essential minerals, especially iodine, it is useful for supporting thyroid function and metabolism.

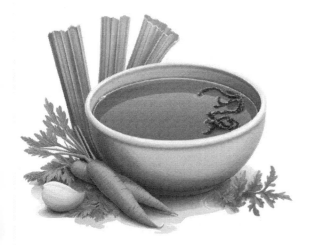

Ingredients:

- 1 tablespoon of dried fucus vesiculosus
- 500 ml of water
- 1 carrot, 1 celery stalk and 1/2 onion
- 1 pinch of whole sea salt

Preparation:

1. Bring the water to a boil with the fucus, vegetables and salt.
2. Let it cook over low heat for 30 minutes.
3. Filter and drink hot as a balancing broth.

Dandelion Purifying Infusion (For Liver & Digestion)

Stimulates liver and digestive function, promoting liver detoxification.

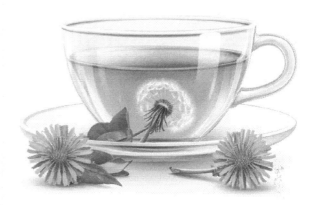

Ingredients:

- 1 tablespoon dried dandelion root
- 250 ml boiling water

Preparation:

1. Place dandelion root in boiling water and let it steep for 10-15 minutes.
2. Filter and drink after meals to aid digestion.

Golden Drink with Ginger (To fight inflammation and improve circulation)

Endowed with powerful anti-inflammatory and digestive properties, it relieves pain and improves circulation.

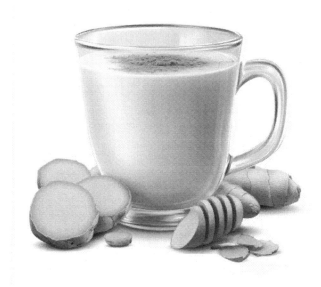

Ingredients:

- 1 teaspoon of grated fresh ginger
- 250 ml sugar-free almond milk
- 1/2 teaspoon turmeric
- 1 teaspoon of honey or agave syrup

Preparation:

1. Heat the almond milk without boiling it.
2. Add the ginger, turmeric and mix.
3. Sweeten with honey and drink before bed.

Licorice Immune Decoction (For the immune system and respiratory tract)

It supports the immune system and has soothing effects on various ailments, especially those related to the respiratory tract.

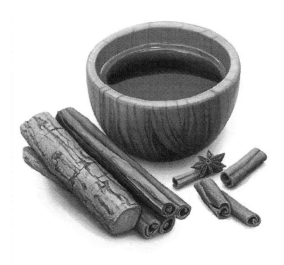

Ingredients:

- 1 teaspoon licorice root
- 250 ml of water
- 1 piece of cinnamon (optional)

Preparation:

1. Boil water, add the licorice root and let it simmer for 10 minutes.
2. Filter and drink when you have a sore throat or feel the first symptoms of a cold.

Relaxing Lavender Infusion (To reduce stress and promote sleep)

Known for its calming and relaxing effect, it is helpful in reducing stress and promoting restful sleep.

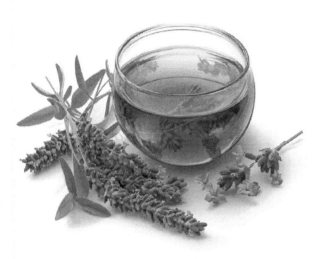

Ingredients:

- 1 tsp dried lavender flowers
- 250 ml boiling water

Preparation:

1. Pour boiling water over the lavender flowers and leave too steep for 10 minutes.
2. Filter and drink before bed to relax.

Red Clover Regenerating Elixir (For Hormonal Health & Vitality)

Aids in cell regeneration and hormonal rebalancing, supporting overall health and vitality.

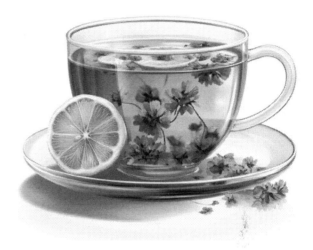

Ingredients:

- 1 tablespoon dried red clover flowers
- 250 ml boiling water
- 1 teaspoon lemon juice

Preparation:

1. Place the clover flowers in boiling water and let it steep for 10 minutes.
2. Strain and add lemon juice to enhance the alkalizing effect.
3. Drink once a day to improve energy and hormonal balance.

PART 2: THE TRANSITION TO AN ALKALINE LIFE

CHAPTER 5: SWITCHING TO THE ALKALINE DIET IN 14 DAYS

Transitioning to an alkaline diet may seem challenging at first glance: abandoning old eating habits and replacing them with a new lifestyle requires determination, patience, and curiosity about what benefits the body. Yet, it is enough to divide this path into well-defined stages to make the change more manageable and sustainable. This chapter focuses on a 14-day program to guide you through transitioning to a diet focused on foods that promote pH balance, reduce inflammation, and boost your body's natural self-healing abilities.

By following the tips in the previous sections, you'll already have an idea of which foods are best suited to promote an alkaline internal environment, as well as the main foods to avoid so as not to generate acidity. However, the real challenge is to transform this theoretical awareness into deep-rooted, long-lasting daily habits. The 14-day method was created with the intention of offering a clear and gradual path, allowing you to concretely experience the benefits of a more natural diet without subjecting your body (and mind) to abrupt changes.

In these two weeks, we will provide practical guidelines and sample menus to help you reorganize your pantry, choose foods in a targeted way, and experiment with new recipes that can satisfy the palate while maintaining a high nutritional profile. You will learn how to properly combine ingredients to maximize the alkalizing effect of meals and reduce inflammatory phenomena that can arise when the body is overloaded with toxins. In addition, we will talk about how to deal with any detoxification symptoms – such as headaches, fatigue, or mood swings – that may occur in the first days of transition and that often discourage those who approach this style for the first time.

One of the most important aspects of this 14-day route is its flexibility. While following a well-defined structure, you will have the freedom to adapt the suggestions to your personal needs, seasonal availability and tastes. This flexibility is designed to make the transition to an alkaline diet less daunting, inspiring you to discover new flavors, creative recipes and smart combinations, all in full respect of your body's needs.

Over the course of these two weeks, you will realize how the alkaline diet is not just a set of rules, but a real lifestyle, in which the harmony between mind and body plays an essential role. In fact, it has been shown that a more conscious food choice positively affects energy, mood and sleep quality, creating a virtuous circle of well-being that is reflected in all aspects of everyday life. This understanding of the benefits of the alkaline diet will motivate you to continue with the transition and adopt it as a long-term lifestyle.

Finally, the 14-day transition represents a springboard toward a more profound change. After this break-in period, it will be easier to continue with a long-term alkaline lifestyle, consolidate the results obtained, and experiment with new recipes and wellness practices. In other words, this chapter marks the beginning of a journey of transformation that does not end at the end of the two weeks but continues with a view to integral health rooted in nature and in harmony with your body.

How to Phase Out Acidic Foods Without Stress

Phasing out stress-free acidic foods means taking a progressive and sustainable approach that allows the body to adapt to changes without suffering sudden trauma or deficiencies. Instead of suddenly giving up all potentially acidifying foods, it is preferable to gradually reduce their quantities and replace them with more alkalizing alternatives. This progressive step helps prevent the sense of deprivation. It allows you to familiarize yourself with new flavors and recipes, keeping your motivation and desire to continue the path high.

The first step is to analyze your eating habits and identify when you most frequently consume unhealthy foods (for example, packaged snacks in the middle of the morning, sugary drinks at lunch, or salty snacks in the afternoon). Once these critical points have been identified, they can be replaced, one at a time, with more natural alternatives: some fruit, a handful of dried fruit, or a homemade bar with whole, unrefined ingredients. Similarly, it is essential to review the main meals, gradually introducing more vegetables, whole grains, and vegetable proteins to reduce the presence of red meats, refined sugars, and industrial products.

The secret to lasting change is to act in small steps: eliminate one particularly acidifying food at a time rather than radically upsetting the diet in a single day. In this way, the body gets used to new balances without being alarmed, and the mind does not perceive change as an unsustainable sacrifice. If you decide, for example, to reduce red meat, you can start by limiting its consumption to only once a week, replacing it with fish or legumes on other days. Similarly, for refined sugars, you can opt for natural sweeteners (such as maple syrup or honey) or sweet fruits, progressively reducing the amount of added sugar in hot drinks and recipes.

Examples of toxic or acidifying foods to be eliminated or drastically reduced

- **Red meats and sausages:** Cured meats, sausages, hams, and processed meats are generally rich in saturated fats and additives.
- **Refined sugars:** Industrial sweets, biscuits, snacks, candies, and sugary drinks.
- **White flour and industrial bakery products:** White bread, crackers, breadsticks, and baked goods made from refined flour and preservatives.
- **Sugary and carbonated drinks:** Soft drinks, energy drinks, fruit juices with added sugar, or chemical sweeteners.
- **Fast and fried foods:** Foods high in trans fats, additives, and salt.
- **High-fat dairy products:** Aged cheeses and butter are often acidifying and challenging to digest.
- **Excess alcohol:** Tough liquor and cocktails with sugary syrups contribute to acidification and liver stress.

- **Convenience and ultra-processed foods:** frozen dishes, instant soups, packaged snacks, and foods rich in preservatives and chemical additives.

Progressively reducing these foods and replacing them with plant-based protein sources, whole grains, seasonal fruits, and vegetables will help keep the body in an optimal acid-base balance. In addition, aromatic herbs, anti-inflammatory spices, and purifying herbal teas will complete the transformation path, making the transition to an alkaline diet smoother and more sustainable.

Numerous scientific studies have shown how the consumption of certain foods can negatively affect health, contributing to the onset of various diseases. Here's an overview based on recent research:

- **Refined sugars:** Although there is no direct evidence linking sugar consumption to increased risk of cancers, excessive intake can lead to overweight and obesity, known risk factors for several types of cancer.
- **White flours and industrial baked goods:** Foods made from refined flours have a high glycemic index, which can cause glycemic and insulinemic spikes. This phenomenon has been associated with an increased risk of cardiovascular complications and could contribute to tumor development.
- **Sugary and carbonated drinks:** Regular consumption of these drinks is linked to an increased risk of obesity and type 2 diabetes. The high content of simple sugars can lead to insulin resistance and inflammation, factors that predispose to chronic diseases.
- **Fast food and fried foods** are often high in trans and saturated fats, which contribute to increased LDL ("bad") cholesterol and the risk of cardiovascular disease. In addition, frying can generate harmful compounds associated with inflammation and oxidative stress.
- **High-fat dairy products:** Excessive consumption of dairy products high in saturated fat can contribute to increased cholesterol and the risk of cardiovascular disease. However, there is no conclusive evidence directly linking dairy products to increased risk of cancers.
- **Excess alcohol:** Even minimal alcohol consumption has been associated with increased cancer risk, suggesting that the healthiest choice is to eliminate it from your diet.
- **Convenience and ultra-processed foods:** A high consumption of ultra-processed foods has been associated with an increased risk of colorectal cancer.

Reducing your intake and favoring a diet rich in fruits, vegetables, whole grains, and plant-based proteins can help maintain optimal acid-base balance and promote long-lasting health.

How to deal with detox symptoms

When you adopt a new, healthier diet and begin to reduce or eliminate acidifying foods, your body can go through a "readjustment" phase during which you experience detoxification symptoms. It is essential to understand that these reactions are completely normal: the body, getting rid of the waste accumulated over time, may show signs of temporary "discomfort," such as fatigue, headaches, irritability, or abdominal bloating. These symptoms, however annoying, represent a physiological step, a deep cleansing that the body implements to regain a healthier balance.

One of the first strategies to deal with this phase is to increase hydration: drinking enough water, perhaps enriched with lemon or purifying herbal teas helps dilute and dispose of toxins more efficiently. It is also essential to give yourself the proper rest: sleep, in fact, is the moment in which the body regenerates and carries out most of the reparative processes. If possible, try to sleep an adequate number of hours and, if you feel the need, give yourself short breaks or moments of relaxation during the day.

Incorporating cleansing herbs into your diet can speed up and facilitate the elimination of toxins. Plants such as dandelion, nettle, and milk thistle support liver and kidney function, promoting the expulsion of waste. Similarly, soothing herbal teas based on chamomile, mallow, or fennel can calm irritation and swelling, helping to restore general well-being. Even moderate physical movement – such as a walk in the fresh air or a light yoga session – helps with circulation and lymphatic drainage, facilitating detoxification.

It is important to remember that these detoxification symptoms are often short-lived. In most cases, they resolve spontaneously within a few days, giving way to a feeling of increased energy and vitality. Once the body has freed itself from the accumulated toxins, it will be able to function more efficiently, with benefits reflected in mood, mental clarity, and physical endurance. Knowing that these reactions are temporary and will lead to positive and lasting results can provide the motivation to overcome the most difficult moments.

Primary symptoms of detoxification and how to manage them

Fatigue and low energy

During detoxification, the body uses extra resources to eliminate accumulated toxins, causing fatigue and a general drop in energy. This happens because the system focuses on purification, subtracting energy from all other daily functions. To address these symptoms, increasing hydration by drinking water regularly is crucial, as the abundant fluid helps to thin out and expel toxins. It integrates purifying herbal teas, such as those made from dandelion, fennel, or other beneficial herbs, which support the liver and kidneys. Give yourself rest breaks throughout the day and choose light physical activity, such as a short walk or stretching sessions, which stimulate circulation and facilitate the work of the body's detoxifying systems.

Headache

The headache that occurs during detoxification can be caused by the sudden release of toxic substances that irritate the nervous system and possible imbalances in hydration levels. This symptom can be exceptionally bothersome, but natural ways exist to relieve it. Drinking plenty of water is essential to restore water balance and promote the elimination of toxins. Reducing caffeine consumption can help prevent further episodes, as caffeine dehydrates the body. Short deep breathing or meditation sessions can also relax the mind, decrease tension, and help reduce headaches naturally.

Irritability and mood swings

During detoxification, eliminating refined sugars and other "comfort" foods can affect levels of serotonin, the hormone that regulates mood, leading to irritability and mood swings. This change can be challenging, but some strategies can help stabilize emotional balance. Incorporate foods into your diet that provide energy consistently, such as fresh fruit, nuts, and whole grains, which release natural sugars slowly into the bloodstream. Set aside time for relaxing practices, such as mindfulness techniques, meditation, or creative activities, that help you reduce emotional stress and maintain a more stable mood during detox.

Abdominal bloating

Abdominal bloating is a common symptom when transitioning to a more natural diet. As gut bacteria adapt to the new diet, they produce excess gas, which can cause discomfort and a feeling of unwanted fullness. To relieve bloating, it is helpful to opt for easily digestible foods and chew slowly, thus allowing the digestive system to work more efficiently. In addition, taking probiotics or lactic ferments can help restore the balance of the intestinal flora, improving digestion and reducing abdominal discomfort.

Feeling nauseous or heavy

A sense of nausea or heaviness can occur during detoxification when the body must quickly eliminate many toxins. This temporary overload can exceptionally affect the liver and kidneys, which must work harder to purify the blood. To manage this symptom, it is advisable to take hepatoprotective herbs such as dandelion and milk thistle, which are known for their support of liver function. In addition, it is essential to listen to your body's satiety signals and opt for light and nutritious meals, avoiding excessive portions that can increase the heaviness, thus allowing the digestive system to function at its best during detoxification.

Remember that these unpleasant symptoms are a natural part of the detoxification process and indicate that your body is working to get rid of the waste. Once this phase is over, you will be able to enjoy a more energetic body, brighter skin, and a clearer mind. The important thing is not to get discouraged. Give the body the necessary time and continue to provide it with the support it needs, both through proper nutrition and healthy lifestyle habits.

Weekly alkaline menu for beginners

The weekly alkaline menu for beginners has been designed to help you transition smoothly to a dietary style that promotes a balanced and less acidifying internal environment. The goal is to combine breakfasts, lunches, dinners, and snacks in a tasty and balanced way that is rich in nutrients, low in sugar, and suitable for those who follow a low-carb diet or are diabetic. By following this plan, you can progressively replace acidifying foods with more natural alternatives, always maintaining an adequate nutritional intake and supporting the body's pH in a favorable range. This menu will provide a concrete example of organizing daily meals, making the transition to the alkaline diet easier, more enjoyable, and more sustainable.

This weekly menu is designed to offer you a solid and flexible starting point: recipes and pairings can be adapted to your personal preferences and the availability of seasonal ingredients. By following this plan, you can gradually get your body used to an alkaline diet, helping to maintain pH balance, improve digestion and support overall well-being, all without excessive sacrifices and with the pleasure of enjoying nutritious and tasty dishes.

Easy-to-make alkaline snacks and drinks

To ease the transition to an alkaline lifestyle, it's crucial to include healthy, easy-to-make, nutrient-dense snacks and beverages in your daily routine. These small food breaks not only provide the energy needed to overcome moments of stress or glycemic drop but also help to keep the level of alkalinity in the body constant, avoiding the use of industrial snacks and sugary drinks that can alter the pH and cause energy fluctuations.

Day	Breakfast	Lunch	Dinner	Snack
Monday	Green smoothie with spinach, cucumber, avocado, lemon and a pinch of ginger, made with unsweetened almond milk	Mixed salad with lettuce, kale, cucumbers, cherry tomatoes and grilled tofu; Dressing: extra virgin olive oil and lemon juice	Mixed vegetable soup (broccoli, cauliflower, spinach) with a steamed white fish fillet	Handful of nuts and pumpkin seeds
Tuesday	Green tea and unsweetened plant-based yogurt with fresh blueberries	Whole wheat quinoa bowl with grilled vegetables (zucchini, peppers, eggplant) and a small coleslaw; Olive oil and lemon dressing	Spinach, avocado and chickpea salad (in small quantities) seasoned with oil and lemon	Celery sticks with homemade hummus
Wednesday	Smoothie with avocado, spinach, cucumber, lemon and vegetable protein (pea powder)	Arugula salad, cherry tomatoes, cucumbers, avocado and smoked salmon; Dressing: extra virgin olive oil and lemon	Baked vegetables (broccoli, cauliflower, carrots) accompanied by marinated and grilled tofu	A portion of fresh blueberries
Thursday	Wholemeal oat porridge with unsweetened almond milk and a small portion of berries	Kale and spinach salad with avocado, nuts and seeds, with olive oil and lemon dressing	Lentil soup with vegetables (celery, carrots, onion) and a portion of green salad	A handful of almonds
Friday	Spinach, avocado, cucumber, lemon and a pinch of turmeric smoothie	Brown rice bowl with mixed vegetables (peppers, zucchini, broccoli) and tofu sautéed in a light tamari-based sauce	Arugula, cherry tomatoes, cucumbers and avocado salad with a small portion of legumes (black beans)	Cabbage and cucumber smoothie with lime
Saturday	Green smoothie with spinach, avocado, cucumber, lemon and chia seeds	Mixed salad with lettuce, rocket, cherry tomatoes, cucumbers, avocado and walnuts; Dressing: extra virgin olive oil and apple cider vinegar	Mixed vegetable soup (cauliflower, broccoli, spinach) with a portion of baked fish (sole or cod)	Baby carrots with hummus

Sunday	Green tea and a small smoothie with spinach, avocado, cucumber and lemon	Quinoa salad with spinach, avocado, cherry tomatoes and sunflower seeds; Dressing: extra virgin olive oil and lemon	Grilled vegetables (peppers, courgettes, aubergines) accompanied by a portion of legumes (lentils) and a sprinkling of aromatic herbs	Handful of mixed walnuts and goji berries

These snacks can be a valuable ally for those who experience busy days or face stressful moments, as they offer essential nutrients, fiber and antioxidants that support the immune system and promote a feeling of well-being. In practice, a well-balanced snack not only satisfies the immediate need for energy but also acts as a support for metabolism and detoxification, contributing to the maintenance of a health-friendly indoor environment.

Green Energy Smoothie

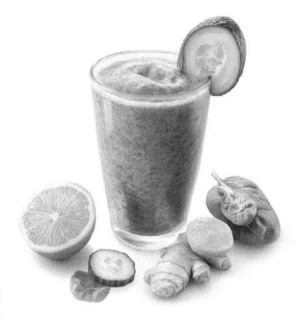

This smoothie is a nutritious drink full of vitality, perfect for starting the day or as a refreshing snack. Make it use a handful of fresh spinach, which provides chlorophyll and vitamins, half an avocado to add healthy fats and creamy texture, half a cucumber that provides hydration and freshness, the juice of half a lemon for an alkalizing touch, and a dash of grated ginger for its anti-inflammatory properties. Top it off with water or unsweetened almond milk and blend until smooth. This smoothie helps you provide your body with natural energy and essential nutrients to support daily well-being.

Fruit and Vegetable Smoothie

Fruit and vegetable smoothie is a great way to obtain a concentrate of vitamins and antioxidants quickly and easily. It uses 2 green apples, which offer a good dose of fiber and vitamins, a cucumber to hydrate and purify the body, a small piece of celery that promotes detoxification and the juice of a lemon for its alkalizing effect. Pass all the ingredients in a centrifuge to obtain a fresh and thirst-quenching juice, ideal for maintaining a good level of hydration and for supporting the body's detoxification processes.

Homemade Bars Made from Seeds and Whole Grains

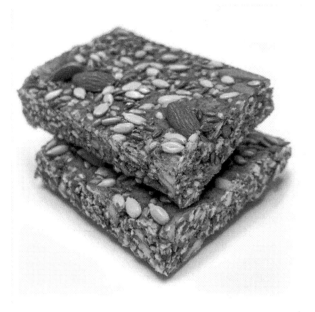

These bars are a practical and nutritious snack that is perfect for taking with you wherever you go. Make a blend with whole grain oats, chia seeds, and pumpkin seeds for a healthy dose of fiber, plant-based protein, and healthy fats, add ground almonds for a crunchy kick, a dash of cinnamon for taste and anti-inflammatory properties, and tie it all together with a natural sweetener like honey or maple syrup, used in small amounts. Mix the ingredients well, spread them on a baking sheet lined with baking paper, press them carefully and bake in the oven at 160°C for about 20 minutes. Once cooled, cut them into bars: they will be a healthy and balanced snack that supports energy throughout the day.

Dandelion Purifying Herbal Tea

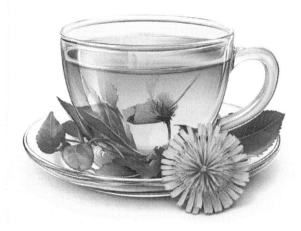

Dandelion purifying herbal tea is a popular natural remedy for supporting liver function and promoting detoxification. Use dried dandelion root, taking about a teaspoon for each cup of boiling water. Leave to infuse for 10 minutes, filter and enjoy the hot herbal tea. This drink helps to stimulate the liver's detoxification system and promote better elimination of toxins, contributing to a more balanced and alkaline interior.

Cucumber and Lemon-Flavored Water

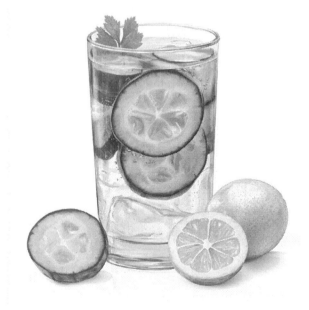

Flavored water is a simple and tasty way to stay hydrated throughout the day, which is essential for supporting pH balance and aiding detoxification. Make this drink by adding cucumber slices and lemon slices to a jug of fresh water, along with a few fresh mint leaves for a fresh kick. Let it sit in the refrigerator for a few hours so that the ingredients release their nutrients and aromas. Not only does this refreshing drink help keep hydration high, but it also helps to create a more alkaline internal environment, supporting the body's overall well-being.

These snacks and drinks not only provide essential nutrients but also act as small "recharge breaks" that help manage stress and prevent energy drops, especially at times when the body needs quick support. Incorporating these simple preparations into your daily routine means offering your body a constant source of clean energy, promoting a feeling of well-being and helping to maintain a balanced internal environment. Over time, these small changes will become a natural habit, contributing to long-lasting well-being and a better quality of life.

The daily routine for a healthy and alkaline life

A healthy daily routine focused on alkaline nutrition is much more than a simple list of habits: it represents an authentic lifestyle that, by integrating proper hydration, movement, stress management techniques, and moments of rest, allows us to live in harmony with our body. Every single action, no matter how small, creates an internal environment conducive to health, helping maintain pH balance and strengthen the body's natural defenses. Imagine starting your day with a calming ritual, such as drinking warm water with lemon. This simple gesture stimulates the digestive system and helps cleanse the body and prepare it for the day's challenges. Continuing, constant attention to movement – which can translate into a short walk in the morning, a few minutes of stretching, or yoga – promotes circulation and lymphatic drainage, key elements to eliminate accumulated toxins and keep energy high.

Stress management is another key aspect. Taking time to practice relaxation techniques, such as meditation or deep breathing, allows us to calm the mind and reduce the internal inflammation that chronic stress can cause. Even short moments of pause during the day, dedicated to a pleasant activity or simply silence, can make a difference, creating a virtuous circle of well-being reflected in all aspects of our lives.

Rest is an essential pillar for consolidating the benefits of a healthy and alkaline life. Quality sleep allows the body to regenerate, repair cells, and strengthen the immune system, while moments of relaxation in the evening help to release the tensions accumulated during the day.

Examples of a healthy daily routine

Morning

Start your day with a glass of warm lemon water. This simple ritual is a natural way to activate the digestive system from the moment you wake up, helping to eliminate toxins accumulated during the night and helping to rebalance the body's pH. Warm water facilitates the mobility of toxins, while lemon, rich in vitamin C and alkalizing properties, stimulates the liver and digestive system. After drinking the water, meditate or do deep breathing exercises for a few minutes. These practices help calm the mind, reduce stress, and increase body awareness, creating a positive mental foundation that promotes emotional and physical balance to face the day's challenges.

1. **Morning break:** In the middle of the morning, when you start to feel a slight drop in energy, take a break to move around a bit outdoors. A short walk or a few stretching exercises stimulate blood circulation but also help release stagnant energy accumulated during sedentary hours. Walking outdoors allows you to breathe fresh air, increase your oxygen supply, and, at the same time, clear your mind. This moment of light movement promotes the release of endorphins, improving mood and preparing the body for a more productive and focused second part of the day.
2. **Lunch:** For lunch, plan a balanced and incredibly alkaline meal, which includes a variety of leafy greens, plant-based protein sources, and whole grains. Such a meal provides a wide range of essential nutrients. It helps keep energy levels stable during the afternoon, avoiding the typical spikes and falls in blood sugar. Eating consciously, without haste, allows the body to assimilate every nutrient optimally and to start the digestive process efficiently. This balanced meal, which also contributes to a more alkaline internal environment, supports overall well-being and helps prevent the buildup of toxins, making the body more resilient to daily stresses.
3. **Afternoon:** In the afternoon, if you notice a drop in energy or a sense of fatigue, treat yourself to a healthy snack to recharge your batteries. A green smoothie, made with ingredients such as spinach, cucumber, celery, and a touch of lemon, offers a combination rich in chlorophyll, vitamins, and minerals, helping to provide energy naturally. Alternatively, a handful of nuts, which provide healthy fats and protein, can be a great option to keep your blood sugar stable. These nutritious snacks are designed to give your body an energy boost without weighing it down, helping you stay focused and prevent feelings of fatigue while maintaining balance throughout the day.
4. **Evening:** The evening is the ideal time to relax and recover from the energy accumulated during the day. Activities such as yoga, meditation, or simply listening to relaxing music can help reduce stress and prepare your mind for rest. At the same time, taking a few minutes to read a good book or take a light walk can help you detach from everyday worries. End the day with a cleansing herbal tea, for example, made from herbs such as dandelion or chamomile, which helps rid the body of toxins accumulated during the day and supports the digestive system, setting the stage for deep and rejuvenating sleep.
5. **Sleep:** Finally, establish a regular nighttime routine that promotes quality rest. Creating a quiet and comfortable environment by reducing exposure to bright lights and electronic devices helps the body release the hormone melatonin, essential for regulating the sleep-wake cycle. Set aside time for relaxing rituals, such as a short meditation or a warm bath, that signal to your body that it's time to slow down. Adequate sleep is essential to allow the body to regenerate, strengthen the immune system, and maintain overall balance in the long run, ensuring that all physiological functions operate at their best the next day.

Adopting these simple daily habits not only helps keep your body's pH in a favorable range but also stimulates vitality, making you more energetic, serene, and fit to face each day. Remember, every little gesture counts, and with constancy, these rituals will become a natural part of your life, bringing lasting benefits and a feeling of deep well-being.

Example 1: Anny, the Stressed Manager

Anna worked as a manager in a large company, spending her days between tight meetings, busy deadlines, and constant phone calls. She was used to having breakfast with a quick coffee, lunch in front of the computer, and ending the day exhausted, often resorting to sugary snacks to cheer herself up. This routine left her increasingly exhausted and irritable, with difficulty concentrating and managing stress.

After inquiring about the benefits of a more alkaline diet, Anna gradually changed her habits. In the morning, instead of the usual coffee, he drank a glass of warm water with lemon to stimulate the purification of the body and rebalance the pH. During the breaks, instead of having another cup of coffee, she allowed herself short walks in the open air: walking and breathing profoundly helped her relax her mind and release muscle tension. It has replaced industrial snacks with natural alternatives, such as a handful of almonds or a green smoothie rich in spinach and cucumber.

In just a few weeks, Anna noticed a marked increase in energy and greater mental clarity. The moments of stress were reduced thanks to his body being less acidic and better able to handle daily pressures. In addition, choosing whole, fiber-rich foods gave her a longer-lasting sense of satiety and a more stable mood. In a short time, Anna felt more vital, more serene, and able to face even the most hectic days calmly.

Example 2: Mark, the Sedentary Worker

Marco worked eight hours daily in the office, sitting at his desk, with very little physical activity. He often ended up eating convenience foods or quick sandwiches. In the evening, he struggled to fall asleep due to prolonged use of electronic devices. The result was a constant sense of fatigue, low productivity, and a fluctuating mood, which was reflected in his private life.

Wanting a change, Marco decided to introduce some simple natural remedies inspired by the concept of the alkaline diet. She started the day with a light but nutritious breakfast, adding fresh fruit, whole grains, and water flavored with lemon and cucumber slices to promote hydration. He got up for stretching exercises or a short walk during work breaks. This slight movement improved circulation and gave him more energy throughout the day.

In the evening, instead of looking at his smartphone until late at night, Marco turned off the screens an hour before sleeping, dedicating himself to a few pages of a book or deep breathing exercises. After a few weeks, he noticed that his sleep quality had significantly improved, as well as his concentration in the morning. By reducing acidic foods (such as sugary drinks and processed foods) and favoring more natural and alkalizing ones (green leafy vegetables, fresh fruit, legumes), Marco has obtained a more stable energy level and a more positive mood, with apparent benefits both at work and in his free time.

Example 3: Sara, the Freelance Mother Struggling with Daily Chaos

Sara, a mother of two children and a freelance worker, dealt with a hectic and disorganized life daily. He often skipped meals or quickly consumed unhealthy foods, resorting to packaged sweets or sugary coffee to compensate for the lack of time. This lifestyle led her to feel constantly fatigued, with digestion problems and frequent mood swings.

When she adopted a weekly menu inspired by the alkaline diet, Sara began to carefully plan her meals, dedicating some time to preparing simple but nutritious dishes. It introduced more raw and cooked vegetables, legumes, and whole grains, progressively reducing refined sugars and processed foods. In addition, she included small moments of mindfulness during the day: short meditation breaks or guided breathing to manage stress.

Within a few weeks, Sara noticed significant changes: digestion improved thanks to a higher intake of fiber and water, while the choice of alkalizing foods helped reduce feelings of heaviness and drops in energy. She also experienced gradual weight loss due to more balanced meals and reduced inflammatory foods. The newfound balance in the diet and the moments of relaxation have allowed her to better manage the daily chaos, restoring serenity and vitality.

CHAPTER 6: DETOX ACCORDING TO DR. SEBI – PURIFYING THE BODY NATURALLY

The concept of "detox" – or purification – has been at the center of countless discussions and approaches to wellness. However, when we talk about detoxification, according to Dr. Sebi, we are referring to a method deeply rooted in the idea that the body possesses extraordinary self-healing abilities and that, if supported correctly, it can rid itself of the waste and toxins that hinder its optimal functioning. This chapter explores Dr. Sebi's vision of natural purification, emphasizing concrete strategies that are easily applicable in everyday life.

Dr. Sebi argued that the accumulation of mucus and toxins was one of the main causes of disease, as it made the biological terrain favorable to the onset of disorders and weakened the immune system. The idea of "intracellular cleansing" – a concept already introduced in previous chapters – finds one of its most significant moments in detox: through a combination of alkalizing foods, purifying herbs, and balanced lifestyle practices, the body is stimulated to progressively eliminate harmful substances, restoring an internal environment that favors the vitality and health of each cell. One of the strengths of Dr. Sebi's method is the holistic approach: detoxification is not seen as a simple fasting or a quick "cure" to lose weight but as an integrated process that involves nutrition, hydration, movement, and stress management. Every aspect of our lifestyle affects the body's ability to cleanse itself. This chapter will show how it is possible to support the body in all its functions, from the most obvious – such as the work of the liver, kidneys, and intestines – to the most subtle, such as regulating acid-base balance and emotional well-being.

This reading will explain how to select the most suitable foods to support the detox process, favoring those rich in alkalizing minerals and those poor in substances that promote inflammation. Indications will be provided on how to integrate specific herbs into one's routine, which can support the work of the excretory organs (liver, kidneys, intestines) and promote the elimination of waste. In addition, some daily practices will be explored – from drinking warm water with lemon as soon as you wake up to breathing and relaxation exercises – which can further facilitate detoxification, making it more fluid and less stressful for the body.

It is important to emphasize that purification, according to Dr. Sebi, is not a drastic or punitive experience but rather an invitation to reconnect with one's body, listening to its signals and offering what it needs. For this reason, space will also be given to advise on managing any detoxification reactions, such as mild headaches or fatigue, remembering that these manifestations often signal that the body is working hard to get rid of what it does not need. With this perspective, detox becomes a journey of awareness and self-care, an opportunity to rediscover the body's inherent wisdom and establish a new relationship with food and nature. In the following paragraphs, practical strategies, recipes, and suggestions inspired by Dr. Sebi's principles will be illustrated in the video, a real handbook to gradually but effectively undertake the road to a deep purification capable of restoring energy, mental clarity and lasting well-being.

The importance of body purification

According to Dr. Sebi's approach, purification is not simply a means to get rid of accumulated toxins but constitutes a real "reset" of the body, an opportunity to restore harmony at the cellular level and promote the full expression of the body's self-healing abilities. The idea behind this concept is that, over time, an unbalanced lifestyle and an unhealthy diet can accumulate mucus and waste, gradually compromising the function of the organs and creating an acidic and inflammatory internal environment.

Getting rid of these residues allows you to experience a feeling of lightness and vitality, as the energy previously used to manage toxins and imbalances is now redirected towards more constructive processes, such as tissue regeneration and strengthening the immune system. In addition, by reducing inflammation and promoting a slightly alkaline pH, a favorable environment is created in which beneficial enzymes and microorganisms can operate at their best, ensuring efficient digestion and better assimilation of nutrients.

From this perspective, purification becomes a fundamental step for those who want to embark on a path of deep well-being: it is not a quick solution or an impromptu remedy but a holistic approach that works on the causes and not just the symptoms. Facing a detox period, in fact, means giving the body a break from negative external stresses, allowing it to regenerate and restore those delicate balances that are often altered by stress, an unbalanced diet, or a hectic routine.

In this way, purification, according to Dr. Sebi, not only gives new energy and mental clarity but also creates the basis for more solid and lasting health, in which the body is better able to defend itself against external aggressions and better support the natural processes of repair and protection.

Dr. Sebi's 7-Day Detox Plan – How to Do It Safely

The 7-day purification plan proposed by Dr. Sebi is designed to purify the body by using alkalizing foods and specific herbs that support the excretory organs, particularly the liver, kidneys, and intestines. The idea is to promote natural detoxification, reduce the intake of acidifying substances, and introduce foods rich in phytonutrients, which favor cell regeneration and overall well-being. To tackle this path safely, you must listen to your body, ensure adequate hydration and consult a qualified professional if you have health conditions. The plan does not involve an abrupt change but a gradual transition: for example, introducing more green leafy vegetables and phasing out refined grains and other processed foods, favoring natural foods rich in beneficial substances.

This 7-day plan, based on a gradual introduction of leafy greens and the phasing out of refined grains and other acidifying foods, aims to give the body a steady source of beneficial phytonutrients. By following this menu, you can give your body the support it needs to cleanse itself safely, promoting effective and lasting detoxification. Each meal is designed to be light yet nutritious, helping to stabilize blood sugar levels and keep energy high, without sacrificing the pleasure of taste and the satisfaction of nutritional needs. With this plan, the transition to an alkaline diet becomes a gradual, sustainable and, above all, rewarding path, which will allow you to experience the benefits of a purified body in perfect balance.

Day	Breakfast	Lunch	Dinner	Snack
Monday	Green smoothie: fresh spinach, cucumber, avocado, lemon juice and coconut water; a handful of chia seeds for extra fiber and antioxidants	Mixed salad: lettuce, spinach, rocket, cucumbers, cherry tomatoes and avocado, seasoned with extra virgin olive oil and lemon juice	Vegetable soup: cauliflower, broccoli and celery, flavored with rosemary and thyme; a serving of grilled tofu to add vegetable protein	A green apple or a handful of nuts
Tuesday	Green tea and a smoothie: kale, green apple, fresh ginger, lemon juice and filtered water	Salad bowl: spinach, kale, cucumbers, peppers and avocado, enriched with pumpkin seeds; Light dressing with olive oil and apple cider vinegar	Warm vegetable salad: zucchini, eggplant, peppers and broccoli sautéed in a pan with a drizzle of olive oil; Side dish of boiled legumes (lentils)	Celery sticks with homemade hummus
Wednesday	Detox smoothie: spinach, kale, cucumber, lemon juice, a pinch of turmeric and coconut water	Arugula and lettuce salad with cherry tomatoes, avocado and sunflower seeds; a splash of lemon juice to enhance the flavors and increase the alkalizing effect	Steamed vegetables: broccoli, cauliflower and spinach seasoned with fresh herbs (rosemary, basil) and a drizzle of olive oil; a portion of marinated and grilled tempeh	Cucumber and mint smoothie
Thursday	Green juice: centrifuged spinach, cucumber, lemon and a piece of ginger	Large salad: lettuce, spinach, arugula, cucumbers, cherry tomatoes, grated carrots and avocado, seasoned with extra virgin olive oil and lemon juice	Mixed vegetable soup: celery, carrots, broccoli and cauliflower, flavored with fresh herbs; Addition of a plant-based protein source such as lightly sautéed seitan	A handful of almonds or walnuts

Friday	Refreshing smoothie: spinach, avocado, cucumber, lime juice and coconut water, with flaxseed for extra omega-3	Bowl detox: Kale, spinach, peppers, cucumber and avocado salad, topped with a dressing of olive oil, lemon and a pinch of black pepper	Grilled vegetable salad: zucchini, eggplant, peppers and broccoli, seasoned with extra virgin olive oil, served with a small portion of legumes (boiled chickpeas)	Purifying dandelion herbal tea, prepared with hot water and a teaspoon of dried herbs
Saturday	Energizing smoothie: spinach, kale, green apple, lemon and coconut water; add a teaspoon of chia seeds	Fresh salad: arugula, lettuce, cucumbers, cherry tomatoes, avocado and pumpkin seeds, seasoned with extra virgin olive oil and lemon juice	Detox soup: pumpkin, cauliflower and spinach with a hint of ginger and turmeric; Side dish of grilled tofu seasoned with herbs	A portion of fresh berries
Sunday	Green tea and a smoothie: kale, spinach, cucumber, lemon juice and filtered water, enriched with a pinch of turmeric and black pepper	Spring salad: lettuce, arugula, spinach, cucumbers, avocado, peppers and cherry tomatoes, seasoned with olive oil and lemon juice	Baked vegetables: broccoli, cauliflower and zucchini, with a drizzle of olive oil and a sprinkling of fresh herbs; side dish of mixed boiled legumes (lentils and chickpeas)	A small green smoothie or carrot sticks with hummus

The role of detox water and herbal teas

Water is an essential element for life and represents the foundation of every biological process in the human body. Every biochemical reaction occurs in a hydrated environment; without adequate water, enzymes and metabolic mechanisms cannot operate efficiently. This vital resource performs numerous fundamental functions: it participates in the digestion and absorption of nutrients, regulates body temperature, facilitates the transport of substances, and eliminates waste products through the liver, kidneys, and skin. For the detoxification process, water acts as a catalyst, promoting the filtration of toxins by the excretory organs and eliminating waste products at the cellular level.

However, the actual value of hydration is not limited to the simple elimination of toxins: proper water intake is essential for energy metabolism and hormonal balance. Drinking water and detox herbal teas regularly helps maintain an optimal metabolic balance and stimulates fat-burning processes. During the fasting state, for example, the body enters a phase of increased metabolic efficiency, using fatty acids as its primary energy source instead of resorting to readily available sugars.

Water-based detox herbal teas play a crucial role in this context, as they do not break metabolic fasting, allowing you to prolong the benefits of lipolysis (the breakdown of fats into energy). In addition, they promote the activation of metabolism and the release of key hormones involved in cell repair and weight management processes. Some compounds present in purifying herbs, such as dandelion, nettle, milk thistle, and fucus vesiculosus, support the liver and kidneys, which are responsible for eliminating toxins and regulating water retention.

Another key benefit of regular consumption of detox herbal teas is their action on the endocrine system, which regulates essential hormones such as insulin, cortisol, and thyroid hormones. Constant hydration with alkalizing herbal teas helps stabilize blood sugar levels, reduce glycemic spikes, and optimize fat metabolism. This process is essential for those who want to lose weight naturally without suffering the adverse effects of overly restrictive diets that often cause hormonal imbalances and slowing metabolism.

Water and herbal teas support thermogenesis, i.e., the production of body heat that contributes to increasing energy expenditure even at rest. Herbs such as ginger, green tea, and cayenne pepper are particularly effective in this regard, as they stimulate calorie consumption and promote the mobilization of fatty acids.

Drinking detox herbal teas several times a day ensures constant purification. It helps prevent subclinical dehydration, which can negatively affect the ability to concentrate vital energy and physical performance. Many people underestimate the impact of chronic dehydration on metabolism. When the body perceives a lack of fluids, it can activate water retention mechanisms and slow down metabolic functions to save energy. This phenomenon can lead to bloating, heaviness, and difficulty burning fat.

Water, therefore, is not only a means of transporting nutrients and facilitating digestion, but it is a genuine activator of metabolism, capable of enhancing fat consumption and improving the body's energy efficiency. Combined with specific herbs, it becomes a powerful tool to promote cellular cleansing, rebalance hormones, and support overall well-being. For these reasons, regular hydration through detox herbal teas is a fundamental habit for anyone who wants to optimize their metabolism, improve the function of the excretory organs, and promote lasting health.

Body hydration

Hydration plays a crucial role in lipid metabolism. Water supports the chemical reactions that break down fats, facilitating their conversion into energy rather than storing them in adipose tissue. Drinking enough, especially between meals, helps maintain an internal environment conducive to the activity of lipid-metabolizing enzymes.

In the morning, as soon as you wake up, the body is back from several hours of rest and needs to replenish fluids to reactivate the metabolism. Water at this stage helps to "wake up" the digestive processes and prepare the body to assimilate nutrients from the first meal. In addition, when you face periods of fasting or go for many hours without food, drinking regularly helps prevent dehydration, support circulation, and optimize the use of fat reserves as a source of energy.

Maintaining a good level of hydration is essential to promote lipid metabolism and ensure a balanced functioning of the whole body, helping to better manage energy and counteract fatigue.

How to prepare and take a purifying herbal tea

To get the most benefit from a cleansing herbal tea, it is essential to use high-quality herbs, preferably organic and stored correctly, to ensure that the active ingredients remain intact and can perform at their best. The preparation of an herbal tea is a simple but powerful ritual: it is recommended to use about a teaspoon of dried herbs for each cup of hot water, leaving to infuse for 5-10 minutes. After filtering the liquid, the herbal tea is ready to be taken. It is essential to vary the types of herbs to amplify the benefits, as each plant offers specific properties. Taking these herbal teas throughout the day, in combination with adequate hydration and a balanced diet, allows you to fully support the body's purification process, contributing both to the cleansing of internal organs and to the support of metabolism, promoting, for example, fat burning and intestinal cleansing.

Milk Thistle Herbal Tea

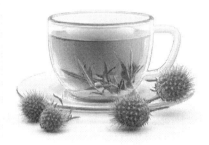

Milk thistle stands out for its protective and regenerating action on liver cells. Its main active compound, silymarin, acts as an antioxidant shield against damage caused by free radicals, thus supporting liver function. A healthy liver is essential for an efficient metabolism, as it participates in the transformation and elimination of many waste substances. Additionally, milk thistle can help improve the lipid profile, helping the body better manage excess fat. This herbal tea, drunk regularly, promotes intestinal purification and supports the immune system, thanks to its anti-inflammatory power and ability to facilitate the regeneration of liver tissues. Also very useful for expelling excess mucus, which Dr. Sebi talked about in his studies.

Ginger and Lemon Herbal Tea

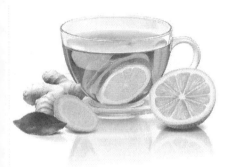

The combination of ginger and lemon is famous for its thermogenic effect, i.e. the ability to slightly increase body temperature and stimulate fat burning. Ginger, in addition to its well-known anti-inflammatory properties, helps calm any digestive discomfort and improve circulation, facilitating the transport of nutrients and oxygen throughout the body. Lemon, on the other hand, is rich in vitamin C and has an alkalizing action, helping to balance the body's pH. This herbal tea is therefore a real panacea for the digestive tract: it reduces swelling, supports the detoxification of the intestines and, thanks to its fresh and pungent taste, can promote a sense of vitality and lightness after meals.

Fennel Herbal Tea

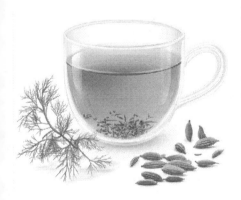

Fennel is characterized by its ability to facilitate digestion, thanks to its essential oils that relax the muscles of the gastrointestinal system. In doing so, it helps reduce abdominal bloating and improve nutrient absorption. In addition to this, this plant is appreciated for its purifying qualities, as it supports the work of the liver and intestines, contributing to the elimination of waste. Fennel herbal tea is also particularly useful for stabilizing blood sugar levels, promoting a more gradual release of energy and preventing blood sugar drops. Also great for finding quick relief when mucus builds up in the airways. Thanks to all these properties, a cup of fennel herbal tea, drunk regularly, can prove to be a valuable ally for the metabolism and for maintaining a healthy and balanced intestinal environment.

CHAPTER 7: NATURAL LIFESTYLE

The natural lifestyle goes far beyond the choice of foods we put on our plates. It is a philosophy that embraces every aspect of our daily lives, inviting us to reconsider our most deep-rooted habits to rediscover a more profound balance between ourselves and our environment. In the previous chapters, we have seen how alkaline nutrition, phytotherapy, and purification can significantly affect health. However, it is time to take a step further and broaden the perspective: a genuinely natural lifestyle does not limit itself to selecting healthy foods. Still, it integrates a series of practices, behaviors, and attentions that complement and consolidate the benefits of a balanced diet.

Think, for example, of physical movement: small changes in our daily habits – such as preferring the stairs to the elevator, dedicating a few minutes a day to simple stretching exercises, or walking in nature – are enough to give the body fundamental support, improving circulation, posture and cardiovascular health. A similar argument applies to stress management, which is often neglected or underestimated but is central to our well-being. Relaxation, meditation, or mindfulness techniques help us calm inner turmoil and promote a psycho-emotional balance, which, in turn, positively impacts the immune system and the body's general functioning.

Similarly, sleep quality plays a crucial role in a 360-degree health journey. Sleeping an adequate number of hours in a quiet environment free of distractions allows the body to regenerate and consolidate the detoxification processes started during the day. The connection with the natural environment also contributes to this picture: dedicating time in contact with nature, whether it is in a city park or a trip out of town, reminds us of our roots and reconnects us with slower and more harmonious rhythms, reducing cortisol levels (the stress hormone) and improving mood.

This chapter, therefore, aims to explore all those practices and attentions that complement and enhance the work done on the food front, transforming the search for well-being into an authentic natural lifestyle. Through practical suggestions and theoretical reflections, we will discover how the choice of cosmetics, home environment care, quality of human relationships, and even free time management can tangibly affect our psycho-physical balance. The goal is to show us how every gesture, however small, can contribute to a more conscious and sustainable existence in which health results from a constant and respectful dialogue between body, mind, and environment.

Adopting a natural lifestyle is not an isolated act or a simple list of rules to follow but a profound choice that stems from the desire to respect our biology and to live in harmony with what surrounds us. Through the following pages, you will have the opportunity to discover how to integrate these practices into your daily routine, experiencing lasting well-being that will reflect not only on your physical fitness but also on your inner serenity and the quality of the relationships you cultivate.

The importance of movement and gentle physical activity

A natural approach to health cannot be separated from movement, as physical activity is one of the most powerful tools to keep the body in balance and promote a good quality of life at any age. Gentle activities – such as yoga, tai chi, or simple walks in the fresh air – are often underestimated but offer extraordinary benefits for overall well-being. These light exercises act on several fronts: they improve blood circulation, stimulate metabolism, help maintain muscle tone, and promote the release of endorphins, the so-called "happiness hormones," which give a pleasant feeling of serenity and fulfillment. In addition, gentle and regular movements help counteract the accumulation of stress, allowing the body to regenerate daily.

The importance of adequate physical activity is particularly evident with advancing age when muscles and joints tend to stiffen, and metabolism can slow down. Even with just a few minutes of light exercise a day, staying active helps prevent muscle loss, preserve bone density, and support cardiovascular health. Regular physical activity also helps stabilize blood sugar levels and support proper hormonal balance, crucial in preventing chronic diseases. In other words, moving constantly, regardless of age or starting conditions, can significantly improve quality of life and longevity.

A concrete example of gentle physical activity within everyone's reach is walking on an empty stomach. This simple habit, preferably done in the morning before breakfast, has several advantages. First, walking on an empty stomach stimulates the body to use fat reserves as an energy source, promoting weight loss and reducing adipose tissue accumulation. In addition, walking on an empty stomach helps regulate insulin levels, avoiding glycemic spikes that can cause fatigue and sudden hunger throughout the day. From a metabolic point of view, morning physical activity optimally activates fat-burning processes. It improves insulin sensitivity, reducing the risk of developing disorders related to altered glucose metabolism.

But that's not all: walking early in the morning, possibly in the open air, allows you to oxygenate the tissues, gradually awaken the body and mind, and start the day with energy and positivity. If practiced regularly, this ritual can turn into a moment of personal reflection, removing stress and promoting concentration for subsequent activities. Integrating walking on an empty stomach into your daily routine, even for just 15-20 minutes, is, a gesture of self-care and an effective way to cultivate deep and lasting well-being.

The Role of Sleep in Healing the Body

Sleep is a fundamental pillar of our health beyond simple physical rest. During sleep, the body enters an active mode of regeneration, in which numerous processes essential for cell repair, hormonal rebalancing, and information processing occur. In the deep stages of sleep – known as slow-wave sleep – the body works intensively to repair damaged tissues, release growth hormones, and stimulate the immune system. This is when cells renew themselves, replacing old or damaged ones with new ones, and when the brain "resets" its connections, consolidating memory and facilitating learning.

Good sleep quality ensures that your immune system is functioning at its best, helping to protect your body from infection and disease. In addition, sleep helps to dispose of toxins accumulated during the day, thanks to the optimal functioning of the lymphatic system and the support offered by cerebral glycolysis. This process cleanses the brain of harmful proteins associated with neurodegenerative conditions.

On the other hand, sleep deprivation or poor-quality rest can impair all these life processes. Lack of restful sleep promotes chronic inflammation, weakens the immune system, and can lead to hormonal imbalances that negatively affect mood, concentration, and even metabolism regulation. Not getting enough sleep exposes the body to a continuous cycle of stress, slowing down the ability to regenerate and making us more vulnerable to illness and ailments.

For these reasons, dedicating the right time and attention to sleep is essential to ensure a complete regeneration of the body and mind. Quality sleep allows you to restore energy, keep vital functions in balance, and prepare the body to face daily challenges with renewed vitality.

How to avoid environmental toxins to protect your health

In addition to what we eat, the environment in which we live plays a crucial role in determining our well-being. Reducing exposure to harmful chemicals is essential to protecting health. For example, choosing cleaning and body care products free of toxic ingredients and opting for natural, untreated materials in our homes helps create a "cleaner" and safer habitat. Good ventilation of environments and the care of green spaces, such as gardens and parks, can also help limit the accumulation of pollutants.

For the person looking for a natural lifestyle and wanting to take care of their well-being in an integrated way, it is also important to go outdoors often. Visiting places surrounded by greenery, where the scent of flowers and natural aromas blend with the fresh air, can make a big difference. City parks, nature reserves, and botanical gardens are ideal spaces to reconnect with nature and recharge your batteries. If you have the opportunity, consider places like the Cinque Terre National Park in Italy, the Gardens of Versailles in France, or large urban parks like Central Park in New York, where the abundance of greenery and the presence of natural elements can create a relaxing and cleansing environment.

These moments of direct contact with nature not only reduce exposure to environmental toxins but also offer psychological benefits: fresh air, bright colors, and the sounds of nature help reduce stress and improve mood, contributing to overall well-being that goes far beyond simple nutrition. Regularly integrating these spaces into your daily life is an effective way to protect your health and live in harmony with the environment around you.

Emotional Well-Being and Positive Relationships

Emotions play a fundamental role in our physical and mental health, directly influencing our well-being. Although we often think of health in terms of nutrition, exercise, and daily habits, our emotional state significantly impacts the body's functions. Stress, anxiety, pent-up anger, and negative emotions can profoundly alter our internal balance, leading to a cascade of physiological effects that undermine our long-term health.

Emotions are not abstract phenomena but neurochemical processes that involve hormones and neurotransmitters. When we experience an intense negative emotion, our body reacts by activating the sympathetic nervous system, releasing cortisol and adrenaline into the bloodstream. This state of alertness is helpful in situations of immediate danger. Still, if it becomes chronic, it can compromise the immune system, increase inflammation levels, and promote the onset of autoimmune and cardiovascular diseases.

Under continuous stress, the body reduces the production of serotonin and dopamine, substances essential for regulating mood and general well-being. This is why a prolonged condition of stress can lead to obvious physical symptoms, such as muscle tension, digestive disorders, chronic fatigue, and difficulty in cellular recovery.

Therefore, learning to manage emotions and improve the quality of one's relationships is essential to maintaining a healthy body and a strong immune system. The first step to achieving this goal is to develop conscious communication, i.e., an interpersonal dialogue based on active listening and expressing one's needs without aggression or repression. Often, relationship conflicts arise not so much from objective differences but from an inability to understand and express one's feelings healthily. Active listening is a practice that allows you to improve the quality of relationships and reduce tensions. Active listening means being fully present during a conversation, avoiding interrupting or mentally formulating a response while the other is speaking. It means observing not only words but also body language, tone of voice, and facial expressions. Communication-based on attentive listening and emotional validation has been shown to reduce cortisol levels and increase the production of oxytocin, the attachment, and trust hormone. When we feel understood and welcomed, our nervous system relaxes, lowering stress levels and creating a condition of widespread well-being.

Another key aspect of emotional well-being is managing one's emotional reactions through regulation techniques. In situations of tension or conflict, it is helpful to adopt strategies that allow you not to react impulsively but to respond more consciously and centered. Deep breathing techniques, meditation, and progressive relaxation can help calm the mind before facing a complex discussion. Teaching your body to get out of the state of excessive activation allows you to reduce the negative impact of stress and maintain control of your emotions.

Developing a positive relationship with yourself is crucial, as well as cultivating a sense of gratitude and appreciation for your life. Gratitude is one of the most powerful emotions for transforming our mental and physiological state. Practicing gratitude daily through simple actions such as keeping a journal where you write down the things you are grateful for has improved mood, reduced stress levels, and increased overall well-being. Gratitude changes how we perceive reality: it helps us focus on what we have instead of what we lack, shifting the focus from problems to available resources. Scientific studies have shown that the practice of regular gratitude has direct effects on the nervous system and brain. On a neurological level, it increases the activity of the prefrontal cortex, the area associated with emotion regulation and positive thinking. On a hormonal level, it stimulates the production of serotonin and dopamine, improving mood and reducing symptoms of anxiety and depression. It has been observed that people who practice gratitude daily have greater emotional resilience and a stronger immune system, as their body is less prone to the harmful effects of chronic stress.

Therefore, integrating emotional well-being into one's life means adopting habits that strengthen our ability to face daily challenges with a more serene and balanced mindset. Positive relationships, practicing gratitude, and developing conscious listening are tools to improve the quality of our social life. They represent fundamental elements of natural health that can positively influence the body and mind. Creating a harmonious relationship environment and cultivating positive emotions reduces stress and inflammation and promotes greater longevity and a lasting sense of well-being.

10. Energy Rituals and Practices for Wellness

Well-being is a matter of nutrition and physical movement and involves the subtle energy surrounding our bodies and spaces. In the holistic tradition, energy rebalancing is fundamental to maintaining a harmonious flow of vitality, reducing stress, and promoting optimal health. Techniques such as aromatherapy, sound baths, and energetic purification of environments are potent tools to restore a profound balance and improve the quality of life.

The use of essential oils for natural healing

Essential oils are one of the oldest forms of natural medicine and have been used for centuries in different cultures to promote physical, mental, and emotional well-being. Extracted from plants, flowers, bark, and roots, these oils contain bioactive compounds that act on the body through smell, skin absorption, and inhalation.

Aromatherapy, or the therapeutic use of essential oils, has been shown to significantly reduce stress, regulate hormones, and improve sleep quality. Oils such as lavender, chamomile, and frankincense are known for their relaxing properties. They can calm the mind, promote deep sleep, and relieve anxiety. Other oils like lemon, eucalyptus, and tea tree have potent antimicrobial properties. They can purify the air and boost the immune system.

The use of essential oils can take place in different ways:

- **Skin Application:** Essential oils can be massaged into the skin to achieve a targeted therapeutic effect when diluted with a carrier oil, such as coconut or sweet almond oil.
- **Aromatic baths:** Adding a few drops of essential oil to the hot bath water promotes muscle and mental relaxation.
- **Direct inhalation** is ideal for essential oils with balsamic effects, such as eucalyptus, which is useful in cases of respiratory congestion.

Essential oils' actions are not only physical but also energetic. Each plant has a vibratory frequency that interacts with our energy field, helping us rebalance our emotions and mental state.

Sound baths with singing bowls and beneficial frequencies

Sound baths are another powerful natural healing tool used to rebalance the body and mind through vibrations. Tibetan singing bowls, gongs, and therapeutic sound frequencies stimulate the release of tensions and energy blockages, promoting a deep state of relaxation and meditation. Each sound frequency has a specific effect on the body and mind. Studies have shown that vibrations produced by instruments such as singing bowls can affect heart rate, blood pressure, and brain waves, inducing a state of relaxation like that of deep meditation.

Sound baths work because our bodies comprise more than 70% water, and water is an excellent conductor of vibrations. When we are immersed in a harmonious sound environment, the vibrations of sound waves resonate with our body, promoting the release of accumulated stress and improving energy circulation.

Energetic cleansing of spaces with incense and sacred herbs

The environments in which we live absorb and retain the energies generated by people, emotions, and events. When space is loaded with stagnant energies, we can feel tired, irritable, or drained for no apparent reason. Energy purification with incense and sacred herbs is a thousand-year-old practice used in many traditions to eliminate negativity and restore harmonious energy.

One of the most powerful tools for energy cleansing is white sage, traditionally used by indigenous North Americans in purification rituals. Smoking salvia can neutralize dense energies and foster a sense of mental and spiritual clarity.

Another widely used plant is palo santo, a sacred wood native to South America, whose smoke is known for its purifying and protective properties. Burning a palo santo stick helps eliminate negative vibrations and create a more serene and harmonious atmosphere.

Rosemary, a plant known for its purifying properties, can also be used to rid rooms of stagnant energy. In ancient times, it was burned in temples and homes to protect against negative influences and increase concentration and mental clarity.

PART 3: PRACTICAL NATURAL REMEDIES FOR HEALING

CHAPTER 8: NATURAL REMEDIES FOR COMMON DISEASES

The use of natural remedies to deal with common diseases has its roots in millenary knowledge, handed down from generation to generation, and today rediscovered with renewed interest by those who want a more holistic approach to health. This chapter explores some of the most effective and safe solutions, drawing on herbal traditions, herbal remedies, and suggestions related to diet and lifestyle. The goal is not to provide miraculous recipes but to offer concrete ideas to gently prevent and manage recurring ailments, respect the body's natural rhythms, and promote the body's self-healing process.

In modern society, we often rely excessively on synthetic drugs, forgetting that nature provides us with an incredible variety of medicinal plants, nutrients, and simple remedies to counteract the most common symptoms, strengthen the immune system, and support general well-being. This approach, strongly supported by Dr. Sebi, is based on the belief that creating an alkaline internal environment and supporting the body's purification systems can solve many health problems without resorting to invasive solutions. Added to this is the idea that each person is a unique system in which body, mind, and spirit interact constantly: for this reason, natural remedies act not only on the symptoms but also on the root causes that may have triggered the disorder.

This chapter will explore some of the most common diseases, such as colds, flu, digestive problems, and joint pain. We will focus on how an alkaline diet, using specific herbs, and adopting healthy habits can help reduce symptoms and speed healing. The most effective foods and medicinal plants, the most suitable preparation methods (such as herbal teas, decoctions, or compresses), and the small precautions that, if applied consistently, can make a difference in recovery and prevention of recurrence, will be highlighted. In addition, we will dedicate a unique space to the importance of stress management and rest, which are often overlooked but fundamental to supporting the immune system and promoting healing.

The natural approach, however, does not exclude conventional medicine, especially in the presence of more complex pathologies; instead, it aims to integrate it and strengthen its effects, improving the quality of life and reducing the need for more invasive interventions. In fact, adopting natural remedies for common diseases does not mean denying the effectiveness of drugs but seeking a balance that allows the body to activate its defense and self-regulation mechanisms, minimizing the side effects and psychophysical stress associated with many conventional therapies.

Natural remedies can be a powerful ally for those who want to live more harmoniously and consciously, cultivating a deep relationship with their body and nature. In the following paragraphs, we will analyze in detail some of the most common disorders, providing practical indications and specific suggestions to deal with them safely and respectfully, as well as the body's physiological processes. The hope is that these pages can inspire a return to ancestral wisdom and, at the same time, promote a modern and integrated vision of health in which every single aspect of our existence – from nutrition to emotions – contributes to creating a lasting balance.

Flu and colds

Digestive disorders, such as bloating, acidity, indigestion, and irregular intestinal transit, can be the result of an unbalanced diet, rich in refined, fried, and highly processed foods. Often, the consumption of acidifying foods such as meat, dairy products and refined flours alters the intestinal microbiota, slowing digestion and increasing inflammation in the gastrointestinal tract. By following the alkaline diet proposed by Dr. Sebi, it is possible to drastically reduce these symptoms through a diet based on natural, fiber-rich and highly digestible foods. The human body functions optimally when it is fed foods that respect its biological balance, avoiding ingredients that produce mucus and inflammation. Dr. Sebi's approach focuses on fresh fruits, leafy greens, alkaline herbs, and non-hybridized grains, all of which promote a more efficient and overload-free digestive process.

In addition to choosing lighter foods, Dr. Sebi's method emphasizes the use of purifying medicinal herbs that support digestion and cleansing of the intestines. Among the most effective are:

- **Fennel:** helps reduce bloating and facilitates the elimination of intestinal gas.
- **Chamomile:** calms gastric inflammation and reduces abdominal spasms.
- **Ginger:** stimulates digestion and accelerates metabolism, preventing fermentation and heaviness.

Another key pillar of the alkaline diet is the promotion of a healthy gut microbiota. While many traditional diets rely on supplementing probiotics through lactic acid bacteria, Dr. Sebi's method focuses on foods that are naturally high in fiber and prebiotics, which feed the beneficial bacteria already present in the gut. These include:

- **Burdock root**, which supports the growth of beneficial probiotic bacteria.
- **Alkaline fruits**, such as figs and dates, which regulate intestinal transit.
- **Bitter vegetables**, such as dandelion and chicory, which stimulate bile production and improve digestion.

Bloating and Constipation

Individuals who struggle with persistent bloating and constipation often benefit from making strategic changes to their daily eating habits. One practical approach is to replace refined starchy foods—such as white bread, pasta, and rice—with non-hybridized whole grains like quinoa or amaranth. These ancient grains provide a higher fiber content, which can help regulate bowel movements and alleviate the sense of heaviness that frequently accompanies bloating. Additionally, incorporating herbal teas made from fennel and nettle can stimulate intestinal transit and support a healthier digestive rhythm. Fennel is known for its carminative properties, which help reduce gas formation. At the same time, nettle can aid in detoxification and gentle diuretic effects. With consistent dietary adjustments over a few weeks, many people notice a rebalancing of the digestive system, leading to less abdominal swelling and improved regularity. Staying adequately hydrated and engaging in moderate physical activity—such as a daily walk—can also enhance these positive outcomes.

Stomach Acid and Reflux

Chronic stomach acid and reflux often stem from lifestyle habits and specific dietary triggers. Coffee, dairy products, and fried foods are common culprits, as they can irritate the esophagus and increase gastric acidity. To counteract these effects, adopting a more alkaline-oriented diet can be highly beneficial. This might include low-sugar fruits (like berries or green apples), leafy green vegetables (such as spinach or kale), and alkalizing seeds (chia and flax), all of which help balance the body's pH levels and reduce acid production. Moreover, eating smaller, more frequent meals and avoiding late-night dining can further lessen reflux episodes. Drinking herbal teas—like chamomile or ginger—may also soothe the stomach lining. Over time, these adjustments often lead to marked improvements in digestion, reducing both the frequency and severity of reflux episodes.

Irritable Bowel

For individuals dealing with Irritable Bowel Syndrome (IBS), processed foods and dairy products can be significant irritants, causing inflammation and discomfort within the gastrointestinal tract. Transitioning to a "cleaner" diet—one that emphasizes fresh vegetables, whole grains, medicinal herbs, and mineral-rich foods—can help calm the intestinal lining and restore a healthier balance in the gut. Adding gentle anti-inflammatory ingredients like turmeric or ginger can further support this healing process. It may also be helpful to identify specific trigger foods through a systematic elimination diet, paying close attention to how certain items (such as high-FODMAP foods) affect symptoms. Coupled with adequate hydration and stress management techniques—like yoga or mindfulness—this approach can markedly reduce flare-ups, improve bowel regularity, and enhance overall digestive comfort.

Following Dr. Sebi's philosophy and adopting an alkaline diet allows you to rebalance the digestive system in a natural way, without resorting to artificial drugs or supplements. Replacing acidifying foods with fresh, nutrient-dense foods not only improves digestion, but also promotes deep detoxification and an overall increase in physical well-being. For those suffering from chronic digestive disorders, this philosophy represents an effective and sustainable solution in the long term.

Joint and Muscle Pain

Joint and muscle pain is often the result of chronic inflammation, the accumulation of toxins in the body, and metabolic imbalances. Many traditional therapies focus on temporary pain management without addressing the root causes of the problem. According to Dr. Sebi's philosophy, however, the real remedy is restoring the body's natural balance through an alkaline diet and purifying toxic residues that fuel inflammatory processes.

Inflammation is the main factor underlying muscle and joint pain. A diet rich in acidifying foods, such as meat, dairy products, refined sugars, and white flour, increases uric acid and free radicals, aggravating inflammatory conditions and slowing down cell regeneration. Dr. Sebi's alkaline diet favors foods that can detoxify the body, reduce excess mucus, and restore an optimal internal pH to counteract these processes. The most suitable foods include green leafy vegetables (spinach, kale, chard), rich in alkalizing minerals and antioxidants, and alkaline fruits (berries, figs, avocado), which provide vitamins and flavonoids for counteracting oxidative damage. Including anti-inflammatory herbs such as nettle, sarsaparilla, and dandelion also promotes the elimination of toxins and blood purification.

Adopting an alkaline diet provides the minerals necessary to strengthen bones and joints. It helps to rebalance the immune system, preventing stiffness and inflammation. According to Dr. Sebi, the natural treatment of muscle and joint pain is based on using medicinal herbs capable of relieving pain and acting on the root causes of inflammation. Among the most effective, sarsaparilla is rich in plant sterols and natural compounds that reduce inflammation and purify the blood, improving circulation at the joint level. Ginger stands out as a natural anti-inflammatory and helps improve mobility. At the same time, thanks to its analgesic properties, turmeric modulates the inflammatory response without the side effects typical of traditional drugs. Finally, the nettle contains minerals such as magnesium and silicon, essential for healthy bones and cartilage. These herbs in herbal teas or decoctions help reduce joint swelling, improve joint lubrication, and combat stiffness and muscle tension. In addition to dietary recommendations and medicinal plants, Dr. Sebi emphasizes the importance of movement to maintain a fluid flow of energy in the body. Moderate physical activity not only improves joint mobility but also stimulates lymphatic circulation, promoting the elimination of toxins and inflammatory substances.

Among the most beneficial practices are alkaline yoga, characterized by gentle movements that improve joint flexibility and reduce muscle tension, and disciplines such as Tai Chi and Qi Gong, which are based on slow and fluid movements that promote relaxation and tissue regeneration. Massages with natural oils, such as arnica or St. John's Wort oil, are also helpful for penetrating deep into the joints and muscles, speeding up recovery processes and relieving stiffness. To further strengthen these effects, combining adequate daily hydration is essential for promoting waste elimination and dedicating time to rest and stress management since sleep and relaxation play a fundamental role in the body's regeneration processes.

Dr. Sebi and the conventional modern lines

The dietary model proposed by Dr. Sebi and the conventional nutritional guidelines share some fundamental principles, such as the importance of an abundant consumption of vegetables and fruit, maintaining a correct intake of vitamins and minerals, and the need to reduce as much as possible excessively processed foods and foods rich in refined sugars. However, Dr. Sebi adopts a much more restrictive approach, eliminating meat, dairy products, and most traditional cereals in favor of alkalizing foods that, according to his philosophy, reduce inflammatory processes and promote healthy bones and joints. On the one hand, this approach can be advantageous for those who suffer from chronic muscle and joint pain since reducing acidosis and taking phytonutrients can help contain systemic inflammation and improve mobility. On the other hand, conventional nutritional guidelines—such as those promoted by research institutions and health organizations—stress a balance that includes animal protein (or well-balanced plant-based alternatives), dairy or sources of calcium and vitamin D, and a variety of whole grains to ensure a complete intake of essential nutrients. Critics of Dr. Sebi's method warn of the risk of nutritional deficiencies, particularly of protein, iron, and B vitamins, especially in the absence of an adequate supplementation plan. At the same time, proponents of the regimen praise its ability to reduce toxic load and excess mucus, which can benefit those struggling with muscle and joint inflammation. Ultimately, choosing between a more rigid regimen and a conventional approach requires an individualized assessment, possibly with the help of a health professional, to balance the goals of reducing pain and inflammation with the need to ensure a proper supply of nutrients for overall well-being.Allergies and Asthma

Allergies and asthma are often the result of an overactivation of the immune system, which overreacts to normally harmless substances such as pollen, dust, mold or certain foods. This state of reactivity is often aggravated by chronic inflammation, acidifying eating, and the accumulation of toxins in the body. Dr. Sebi's philosophy and his alkaline diet represent an effective approach to rebalance the immune system, reduce inflammation and support the body in better managing allergic and respiratory reactions. The first step in reducing the body's reactivity to allergens is to eliminate acidifying foods that overload the immune system and increase mucus production in the respiratory tract. Foods such as dairy, refined sugars, processed foods, and white flours promote an acidic internal environment, which weakens the body and makes it more vulnerable to inflammatory reactions.

Dr. Sebi's alkaline diet, on the other hand, promotes the consumption of foods rich in minerals, antioxidants and anti-inflammatory compounds, which are essential for strengthening natural defenses and reducing the production of histamine, the chemical responsible for allergic reactions.

Natural Management of Allergies and Asthma

According to Dr. Sebi's philosophy, the use of medicinal herbs is essential to help the body detoxify, reduce inflammation, and improve lung function. Several natural remedies act specifically on the respiratory system: licorice root, for example, works like a natural cortisone, reducing inflammation of the respiratory tract and improving breathing; nettle, rich in natural antihistamines, helps contain allergic reactions; fenugreek promotes the elimination of excess mucus from the lungs and alleviates bronchial irritation; Finally, ginger and turmeric have an effective anti-inflammatory action, limiting mucus production and supporting respiratory capacity. Regular intake of herbal teas based on these herbs can be a valid remedy to prevent allergic crises and improve lung health in the long run. In parallel, it is essential to reduce exposure to environmental allergens such as mold, dust, and chemicals, which can aggravate allergies and respiratory disorders. The use of air purifiers, the use of natural fabrics for bedding and clothes, avoiding synthetic materials that trap dust and irritants, and the diffusion of essential oils such as eucalyptus and thyme, which can purify the air and make breathing easier, are all useful strategies to create a cleaner, toxin-free environment. In this way, the frequency and intensity of allergic reactions are reduced, facilitating smoother breathing and greater overall well-being. Dr. Sebi emphasized how an organism free from excess mucus and irritants could react more effectively to external stimuli, preventing acute episodes of allergy or asthma and significantly improving the quality of life.

Concrete Examples of Healing Through the Alkaline Diet

Seasonal Allergies (Allergic Rhinitis)

An individual suffering from seasonal allergies or allergic rhinitis can often benefit significantly from reducing or eliminating dairy products and refined sugars. These foods exacerbate inflammation and increase mucus production, intensifying allergic symptoms. Replacing them with nettle tea, quercetin-rich fruits (such as apples, berries, and grapes), and green vegetables provides the body with powerful antioxidants and bioflavonoids that help modulate the immune response. Nettle has long been used in herbal medicine to reduce histamine levels and alleviate congestion. At the same time, quercetin can stabilize the cells responsible for releasing histamine, easing common symptoms like sneezing, runny nose, and itchy eyes. Over a few weeks, many people notice that these dietary changes contribute to a more balanced immune system and a noticeable reduction in allergy flare-ups.

Chronic Asthma

For someone with chronic asthma, introducing fenugreek, licorice root, and ginger into daily meals or through herbal teas can make a considerable difference in respiratory health. Fenugreek seeds are traditionally known to help clear excess mucus from the respiratory tract. At the same time, licorice root possesses soothing and anti-inflammatory properties that can reduce irritation in the bronchial tubes. Ginger, a well-known natural anti-inflammatory, supports healthy circulation and can help relax the airway muscles, easing breathing difficulties. By simultaneously eliminating or reducing foods that tend to trigger mucus production—often dairy, processed sugars, and certain refined grains—many individuals experience improved respiratory capacity. Over time, these dietary adjustments may lead to fewer asthma attacks and a decreased reliance on bronchodilator medications. However, it is important to continue following any prescribed medical treatment.

Allergic Dermatitis

Skin allergies and dermatitis frequently stem from underlying inflammation within the body. Adopting a diet that emphasizes alkaline and antioxidant-rich foods—such as leafy green vegetables, fresh fruits, and certain nuts or seeds—helps combat this inflammation at its source. Alkaline foods support the body's natural pH balance, leading to more efficient detoxification. At the same time, antioxidants help neutralize free radicals that can aggravate skin conditions. Adequate hydration and including healthy fats (like those found in avocados and cold-pressed oils) further support the skin's barrier function, reducing dryness, itching, and irritation. In many cases, these dietary adjustments lead to visibly calmer, healthier skin and significantly reduce the frequency and severity of dermatitis flare-ups.

Allergies and asthma are not isolated problems, but signs of a body overloaded with toxins and an overactive immune system. Following Dr. Sebi's alkaline diet, rich in anti-inflammatory and purifying foods, combined with the use of the right medicinal herbs and care of the home environment, represents an effective and natural solution to significantly reduce symptoms and improve quality of life.

This approach not only relieves symptoms, but works at the root of the problem, strengthening the body and preventing future allergic or respiratory reactions.

Insomnia and Stress

Insomnia and chronic stress are two of the most prevalent problems in modern society, often underestimated despite their devastating impact on physical and mental health. Lack of sleep and constant tension alter hormone production, weaken the immune system and promote silent inflammatory processes that can degenerate into chronic diseases. Conventional medicine tends to treat these disorders with drugs that are often addictive and mask the problem without solving the causes. Dr . Sebi's philosophy, on the other hand, offers a natural and sustainable approach to rebalancing the body and mind through an alkaline diet, the use of relaxing herbs and energy wellness practices.

Stress and insomnia are strongly influenced by the body's acidic state. When the body is overloaded with toxins, refined sugars, and processed foods, the nervous system remains in a state of overactivation, preventing natural relaxation and disrupting the production of melatonin and serotonin, two hormones key to sleep and emotional well-being.

Following an alkaline and anti-inflammatory diet helps balance the nervous system, improve sleep quality and reduce the production of cortisol, the stress hormone. Some of the best alkaline foods to combat insomnia and stress include:

- Fruits rich in magnesium (**avocados**, **figs**, **bananas**): promote muscle relaxation and serotonin production.
- Green leafy vegetables (**spinach**, **kale**, **chard**): alkalize the body and reduce acidity that alters the nervous system.
- Alkalizing seeds (**pumpkin seeds**, **chia seeds**): rich in tryptophan, an amino acid precursor of melatonin.

The alkaline diet helps to rebalance neurotransmitters, reducing irritability, anxiety and difficulty falling asleep. In addition, eliminating exciting foods such as caffeine, refined sugars and white flours helps to keep your energy level stable during the day and improve your night's rest.

Herbs and Natural Remedies

Medicinal herbs are a key element in Dr. Sebi's philosophy, as they offer natural support to calm the nervous system without side effects. Some herbs that are particularly effective for insomnia and stress include:

Lavender, valerian, passionflower, linden, and **chamomile** are five medicinal plants beneficial for insomnia or sleep-related disorders, thanks to their relaxing and calming properties that naturally act on the nervous system. For example, Lavender (Lavandula angustifolia) owes its effectiveness to the high content of linalool and linalyl acetate, two active ingredients capable of reducing anxiety and nervous tension, promoting gradual and deep relaxation without interfering with normal metabolic processes. Valerian root (Valeriana officinalis) is rich in valerianic acids and other compounds that, by modulating the availability of GABA (gamma-aminobutyric acid, one of the primary inhibitory neurotransmitters of the central nervous system), promote more profound and better-quality rest, without altering the natural sleep-wake cycle. Passionflower (Passiflora incarnata) contains alkaloids and flavonoids—including chrysin—that help regulate the nervous system's activity, reducing mental hyperactivity and promoting gentle muscle relaxation. Linden (Tilia platyphyllos or Tilia cordata), commonly known as linden, owes its relaxing properties to mucilage, essential oils, and flavonoids that synergize to reduce psychophysical tension and facilitate evening relaxation. Finally, chamomile (Matricaria chamomilla) contains apigenin, bisabolol, and other compounds that, in addition to having a soothing effect on the nervous system, calm any digestive disorders that often contribute to insomnia. These plants integrate harmoniously into the body's metabolism since their active ingredients act gently and gradually without causing addiction or side effects typical of some sedative drugs. This way, they promote a more restful and lasting sleep while respecting the body's physiological rhythms. Consuming evening herbal teas based on these herbs helps prepare the body for sleep and reduce the activation of the sympathetic nervous system, promoting a state of calm and relaxation.

Another fundamental aspect to improve sleep and reduce stress is the environment in which you sleep and live. Stagnant energy, electromagnetic pollution, and disharmonious vibrations can interfere with rest.

Creating a clean and balanced sleeping space promotes deep and restful sleep, improving cell regeneration and mental well-being.

1. **Case of Chronic Insomnia:** An individual who struggles to fall asleep could eliminate coffee and refined sugars, replacing them with a light dinner of alkalizing vegetables and a relaxing chamomile and valerian herbal tea. After a few weeks, the quality of sleep improves significantly.
2. **Case of Nocturnal Awakenings and Stress:** Those who wake up frequently during the night can benefit from the use of natural magnesium found in pumpkin and fig seeds, combined with breathing techniques to reduce cortisol. This combination helps to maintain deep and continuous sleep.
3. **Case of Daytime Stress and Anxiety:** A person with high levels of stress and nervous tension could integrate passionflower infusions and meditation with lavender essential oils into their daily routine, significantly reducing states of agitation and promoting greater serenity.

Insomnia and stress are not problems to be underestimated, as they have a direct impact on physical and mental health. Dr. Sebi's philosophy offers a natural and sustainable approach, based on an alkaline diet, the use of relaxing herbs and care for the environment, to rebalance the body and promote a regenerating rest.

Following these principles allows you to improve the quality of life in a profound and lasting way, without resorting to chemical drugs or temporary solutions. Sleeping well means living better, with more energy, mental clarity and overall well-being.

PART 4:
CHRONIC DISEASES

CHAPTER 9: DR SEBI AND DIABETES

Diabetes management is one of the most common and complex challenges in modern society. Today, where the diet is often characterized by excess refined sugars, saturated fats, and processed foods, blood sugar levels tend to rise and remain constantly high, causing both short- and long-term complications. This condition, if not managed properly, can lead to serious cardiovascular, renal, nervous, and even visual damage, threatening quality and lifespan.

A particularly worrying aspect is the increase in type II diabetes among children. This phenomenon reflects the radical change in the eating habits of the new generations. Young people are increasingly exposed to unbalanced diets that are rich in processed foods and low in nutrients, a dietary pattern transmitted directly by parents or educators. This poor diet, combined with a sedentary lifestyle, has led to an alarming increase in cases of childhood diabetes, making this disease a truly terrible public health problem.

In this scenario, a holistic approach that includes an alkaline diet, herbal remedies, and adopting healthy daily habits emerges as an effective strategy for containing and managing diabetes. This approach is not limited to correcting the diet. Still, it aims to restore an overall balance in the body, promoting better insulin sensitivity and more efficient blood sugar regulation. Integrating conscious food choices, practicing regular physical activity, and using specific medicinal herbs allows you to support the metabolism naturally, helping to reduce inflammation and prevent the complications typical of diabetes.

While diabetes continues to threaten the health of millions of people, especially in an age when even the youngest are affected, it is crucial to promote lifestyles that prioritize holistic well-being. Adopting an alkaline diet, supported by natural remedies and healthy daily habits, can be a valid alternative to improve the quality of life, offering concrete hope in the fight against a disease that, if neglected, can have devastating consequences.

Refined sugars and acidity in the body

Prolonged and uncontrolled consumption of refined sugars, such as sucrose and syrups with a high fructose content, is one of the main risk factors for the development of prediabetic states and diabetes. When these sugars are ingested, they quickly enter the bloodstream, causing glycemic spikes that force the pancreas to secrete large amounts of insulin to bring glucose values back to normal. Over time, this mechanism becomes fatigued, and the pancreas loses efficiency, leading to reduced insulin sensitivity and a progressive worsening of glycemic control.

In addition to the direct impact on blood sugar, a diet rich in refined sugars increases the acid load in the body. Industrial foods and foods with a high glycemic index tend to leave acidifying residues, which the body struggles to neutralize if they are not balanced by an adequate intake of alkaline foods. This excess acidity, over time, can trigger a chronic inflammatory state, which not only worsens insulin sensitivity but also promotes the development of other metabolic diseases such as obesity, cardiovascular disease, and osteoporosis.

Chronic acidosis is self-reinforcing: the high level of acidity in the body induces further inflammation and oxidative stress, which further impair the cells' functioning and the immune system's ability to respond to toxins. This harmful cycle is already established during pre-adulthood when incorrect eating habits begin to make their way and progressively worsen until old age. Young people who regularly consume foods rich in refined sugars risk developing an unstable metabolic base, which, over the years, can result in serious diseases, such as diabetes, cardiovascular problems, and even alterations in bone density. Controlling the intake of refined sugars and industrial products is crucial for preventing the accumulation of acidity in the body, breaking the vicious cycle of chronic inflammation, and preserving metabolic health in the long term. Adopting a diet that favors alkaline and natural foods, along with an active lifestyle and stress management practices, is essential in counteracting these effects and improving the quality of life from youth to old age.

How Alkaline Nutrition Helps Stabilize Blood Sugar

An alkaline diet favors plant-based foods, such as green leafy vegetables, fresh fruits, legumes, and whole grains, which offer a low glycemic load and a high content of fiber, essential vitamins, and minerals. These foods provide energy in a balanced way and help maintain a more balanced internal pH, limiting the production of acid waste. A less acidic internal environment is conducive to reducing the underlying inflammatory state, which often impairs insulin efficiency and contributes to harmful glycemic fluctuations.

Green leafy vegetables such as spinach, Swiss chard, and kale, along with vegetables such as zucchini, cucumber, and bell peppers, are rich in fiber that slows down the absorption of sugar into the blood, helping to avoid sudden spikes in blood sugar and ensures a more gradual release of energy. In addition, these foods contain numerous micronutrients that support metabolism and strengthen the immune system. Foods such as avocado and almonds, rich in healthy fats, help to prolong the feeling of satiety, thus reducing the temptation of sugary or low-nutrient snacks and promoting a constant energy balance throughout the day.

Dr. Sebi's philosophy is particularly successful in this context. He advocated the importance of an all-natural, alkaline diet to restore internal harmony and promote the body's self-healing. By following its principles, the symptoms related to glycemic imbalance are alleviated, and the inflammatory roots of diabetes are also counteracted. A diet based on whole, unprocessed foods, rich in nutrients and low in refined sugars, helps stabilize blood sugar, improving insulin sensitivity and reducing the risk of metabolic complications.

This approach means investing in a lifestyle that promotes well-being and vitality, reducing oxidative stress and chronic inflammation that often accompanies diabetes. Natural foods nourish the body and act as preventive medicine, helping to maintain internal balance and prevent the onset of chronic diseases. Dr. Sebi's philosophy, therefore, is based on the idea that giving back to the body what nature offers in a pure and unaltered form can lead to a better quality of life, with relieved symptoms, a more efficient metabolism, and a more incredible feeling of general well-being.

Several scientific studies have shown that a higher intake of vegetable fibers can significantly reduce excess sugars in the body and improve general, physical, motor, and psychophysical health. Fibers, divided into soluble and insoluble, play a crucial role in slowing down the absorption of carbohydrates, helping to avoid glycemic peaks and promoting a more gradual release of energy.

A study published in the *American Journal of Clinical Nutrition* has shown that increasing the intake of soluble fiber in foods such as legumes, oats, and fruit significantly reduces postprandial glucose levels. Soluble fiber forms a gel in the stomach and intestines, slowing down the digestion and absorption of carbohydrates. This mechanism stabilizes blood sugar and helps improve insulin sensitivity, reducing the risk of developing insulin resistance, a precursor condition to type II diabetes.

Other studies published in journals such as the *British Journal of Nutrition* show that a diet rich in vegetable fiber positively influences intestinal microbiota composition. A balanced microbiota is associated with better metabolism regulation and a more extraordinary ability of the body to process and use glucose efficiently. This interaction between fiber and gut flora supports glycemic control. It promotes physical and motor health benefits, thanks to improved digestive function and increased energy for daily activity.

Regular fiber intake is also linked to improved mental and physical health. Fiber helps maintain a feeling of fullness that can prevent excessive intake of high-GI foods, thereby reducing anxiety and mood swings associated with rapid spikes and dips in blood sugar. In behavioral nutrition studies, it has been found that a high-fiber diet is related to a better quality of life and a reduction in symptoms of stress and depression, as a more stable metabolism also has positive effects on brain function and mood. Numerous studies suggest that a high intake of plant fiber contributes to better overall physical health. Increasing the consumption of vegetables, fruits, legumes, and whole grains not only reduces the glycemic load and the risk of diabetes but also promotes weight loss, improves cardiovascular function, and promotes joint mobility, which is essential for maintaining a good level of motor activity.

Effects of Glycemic Index Control

A diet based on foods with a low glycemic index is fundamental in maintaining stable blood sugar control. Foods with a low glycemic index release glucose into the blood gradually, avoiding sharp peaks and falls that can lead to insulin resistance and long-term complications. Numerous studies, published, for example, in the *American Journal of Clinical Nutrition*, have shown that regular intake of whole grains, legumes, and vegetables, all characterized by a low glycemic index, helps improve insulin sensitivity and reduce the risk of developing type II diabetes. But it also helps prevent microvascular and macrovascular damage, which are among the most serious complications of diabetes, such as cardiovascular disease and neuropathy. The beneficial effect also extends to energy metabolism, as a gradual release of sugars allows a constant supply of energy to the cells, avoiding overloading the system and promoting more efficient management of fat reserves.

Adopting a low-glycemic index diet is a strategic intervention for the prevention and management of diabetes. It helps to improve not only metabolic health but also quality of life in the long term.

Interaction between gut microbiota and metabolism

The intestinal microbiota, i.e., the set of microorganisms that inhabit our intestine, has a decisive impact on metabolism and blood sugar regulation. Regular dietary fiber intake, typical of a diet rich in plant and whole foods, is essential to promote the development of a balanced intestinal flora. Studies published in the *British Journal of Nutrition* and other scientific journals have shown that a diet rich in fiber not only improves intestinal transit but also promotes the production of short-chain fatty acids, in particular butyrate. Butyrate has significant anti-inflammatory properties and plays a key role in improving the function of intestinal cells, strengthening the mucosal barrier, and contributing to more efficient absorption of nutrients. In addition, this metabolite modulates the insulin response, contributing to better management of blood glucose levels. A healthy microbiota is, therefore, related to increased insulin sensitivity and a reduced risk of developing metabolic disorders.

Further research, such as that conducted in behavioral nutrition and metabolomics, underlines that a balanced intestinal composition promotes synergy between the nutrients taken and cellular functions, extending the benefits on a psychophysical level. Improving the health of the gut microbiota by increasing the intake of fiber and plant foods can help reduce systemic inflammation, regulate carbohydrate metabolism, and improve overall well-being, thus creating a virtuous cycle that supports the body in managing blood sugar levels and eliminating toxins. The positive interaction between a high-fiber diet, the health of the gut microbiota, and metabolism is a fundamental pillar in preventing and managing diseases such as diabetes, with tangible physical and psychophysical benefits. This holistic approach, which integrates conscious food choices and gut flora support, can significantly contribute to improving quality of life.

The best herbs to balance blood sugar levels

Thanks to their natural properties, some medicinal plants have proven particularly effective in regulating blood sugar. When integrated into a balanced diet and healthy lifestyle, these herbs can significantly support modulating blood glucose levels, reducing glycemic spikes, and improving insulin sensitivity. It is important to emphasize that although these herbs can complement medical therapies, they should not replace treatments prescribed by health professionals.

Gymnema Sylvestre

Known as the "sugar destroyer," Gymnema Sylvestre is a traditional herb used in Ayurvedic medicine for centuries to control blood sugar. Its active compounds, such as gymnemic acids, temporarily inhibit sweet taste receptors, thus reducing cravings for sugars and sweets. Additionally, scientific studies suggest that this plant may stimulate beta cells in the pancreas, promoting more effective modulation of insulin production and helping to stabilize blood glucose levels. Integrating Gymnema Sylvestre into the diet can, be a valuable ally in reducing post-meal glycemic spikes and maintaining more constant glycemic control over time.

Cinnamon

Cinnamon is more than just an aromatic spice: it has powerful hypoglycemic properties. Several studies have shown that cinnamon, thanks to its bioactive compounds such as cinnamaldehyde, improves insulin sensitivity and slows down the absorption of carbohydrates in the intestine. These combined effects help reduce blood glucose spikes after meals, stabilizing sugar levels and improving diabetes management. Regular intake of cinnamon may also have a protective effect on the cardiovascular system, reducing LDL cholesterol levels and improving overall health.

Ginseng (Panax ginseng)

Ginseng, especially Panax ginseng, is one of the most prized herbs for its adaptogenic properties. This means it helps the body respond to stress by modulating the endocrine system and improving its ability to regulate glucose levels. Numerous studies have shown that ginseng can improve carbohydrate metabolism by increasing insulin sensitivity and reducing blood sugar levels. Its stimulating properties, besides providing energy, also promote overall well-being, supporting cognitive function and physical endurance.

Fenugreek

Fenugreek is rich in soluble fiber, which plays a key role in slowing down the absorption of carbohydrates, thus preventing abrupt increases in blood sugar. The active compounds found in this plant, such as saponins, improve insulin sensitivity and promote more stable glycemic control. In addition, fenugreek is known for its beneficial effect on digestion and its ability to increase feelings of fullness, helping to reduce the intake of foods high in sugar. These benefits make it a valuable support for those trying to manage diabetes naturally, effectively supplementing the diet with an ally that promotes glucose regulation and overall metabolic well-being.

Each of these herbs offers a unique and complementary contribution to managing blood sugar levels. By integrating them into a balanced diet and a healthy lifestyle, you can significantly improve glycemic control and reduce the risk of complications associated with diabetes. These herbs, when used in support of traditional therapies, can contribute to a more natural and sustainable management of the disease, promoting a better quality of life and a higher overall well-being.

Smoothies and alkaline recipes for diabetes

Classic Green Smoothie

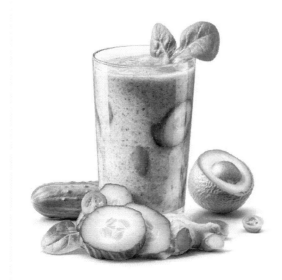

Prep Time: 5 min,

Ingredients:

- 1 handful of fresh spinach
- 1/2 cucumber
- 1/2 avocado
- 1 pinch of grated ginger
- 200 ml of water or unsweetened almond milk

Instructions:

1. Wash the spinach and cucumber thoroughly.
2. Cut the cucumber and avocado into pieces.
3. Put all the ingredients in the blender, add ginger and the chosen liquid.
4. Blend until smooth.

Celery, Green Apple and Lemon Smoothie

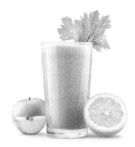

Ingredients:

- 2 stalks of celery
- 1 green apple
- Juice of 1/2 lemon
- 200 ml coconut water

Instructions:
1. Wash the celery stalks and the green apple.
2. Cut the apple into pieces, removing the core.
3. Blend the celery, apple and lemon juice with the coconut water.
4. Strain if you prefer a smoother consistency

Kale and Cucumber Smoothie

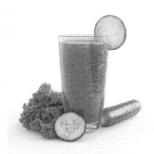

Ingredients:

- 1 handful of kale
- 1/2 cucumber
- 1/2 avocado
- A few fresh mint leaves
- 200 ml of water

Instructions:
1. Wash the kale, cucumber and mint.
2. Remove the stems from the cabbage and cut the cucumber and avocado into pieces. Blend

Broccoli and Spinach Smoothie

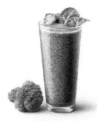

Ingredients:

- 1 small portion of raw broccoli (about 100 g)
- 1 handful of fresh spinach
- 1/2 cucumber
- Juice of 1/2 lemon
- 200 ml coconut water

Instructions:
1. Wash the broccoli, spinach, and cucumber.
2. Cut the cucumber into pieces and separate the florets from the broccoli.
3. Blend all the ingredients together with the lemon juice and coconut water.

Ginger, Lime and Mint Smoothie

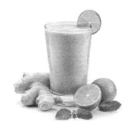

Ingredients:

- 1 small piece of fresh ginger (approx. 1 cm)
- Juice of 1 lime
- 5-6 fresh mint leaves
- 200 ml filtered water

Instructions:

1. Peel the ginger and cut it into small pieces.
2. Squeeze the lime to get the juice.
3. Put the ginger, lime juice and mint leaves in the blender with the water. Blend.

Fennel and Green Apple Smoothie

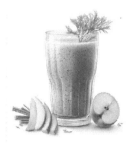

Ingredients:

- 1 small fennel
- 1 green apple
- 1/2 cucumber
- Juice of 1/2 lemon
- 200 ml of water

Instructions:

1. Wash the fennel, apple and cucumber.
2. Cut the fennel and cucumber into pieces; Remove the core from the apple and cut it into slices.
3. Blend all the ingredients with the lemon juice and water until smooth.

Carrot and Turmeric Smoothie

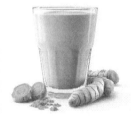

Ingredients:

- 2 medium carrots
- 1 piece of fresh ginger (1 cm)
- 1/2 teaspoon turmeric powder
- 200 ml unsweetened almond milk

Instructions:

1. Wash and peel the carrots; cut them into pieces.
2. Peel the ginger and chop it finely.
3. Place the carrots, ginger, turmeric and almond milk in the blender. Blend.

Avocado and Black Pepper Smoothie

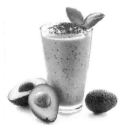

Ingredients:

- 1/2 avocado
- 1 handful of spinach
- 1/2 cucumber
- A pinch of black pepper
- 200 ml coconut water

Instructions:

1. Wash the spinach and cucumber; Cut the cucumber into pieces.
2. Cut the avocado in half and remove the pit.
3. Put all the ingredients in the blender, add a pinch of black pepper and coconut water. Blend

Tomato and Basil Smoothie

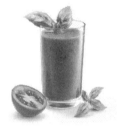

Ingredients:

- 1 ripe tomato
- 1 handful of fresh basil
- 1/2 cucumber
- Juice of 1/2 lemon
- 200 ml of fresh water

Instructions:

1. Wash the tomato, cucumber and basil.
2. Cut the tomato and cucumber into pieces.
3. Blend all the ingredients together with the lemon juice and water until smooth.

Celery, Tomato and Lemon Smoothie

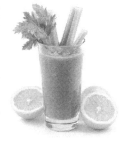

Ingredients:

- 2 stalks of celery
- 1 tomato
- Juice of 1/2 lemon
- A handful of parsley
- 200 ml of water

Instructions:

1. Wash the celery, tomato and parsley.
2. Cut the celery and tomato into pieces.
3. Blend all the ingredients with the lemon juice and water until smooth.
4. Serve chilled for an immediate detoxifying effect.

Spinach, Cucumber and Kiwi Smoothie

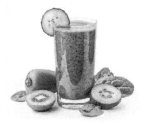

Ingredients:

- 1 handful of spinach
- 1/2 cucumber
- 1 kiwi
- 200 ml coconut water

5.

Instructions:

1. Wash the spinach and cucumber; Peel the kiwi and cut it into pieces.
2. Put all the ingredients in the blender along with the coconut water.
3. Blend until smooth.

Ginger, Celery and Lime Smoothie

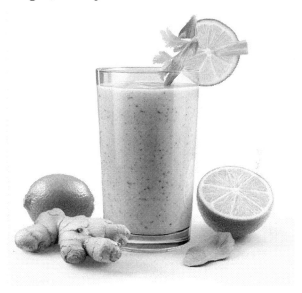

Prep Time: 5 min,

Ingredients:

- 1 piece of fresh ginger (approx. 1 cm)
- 2 stalks of celery
- Juice of 1 lime
- 200 ml filtered water

Instructions:

1. Peel the ginger and cut it into small pieces.
2. Wash the celery and cut it into pieces.
3. Squeeze the lime to get the juice.
4. Blend the ginger, celery, lime juice and water until smooth.

Exercises and daily habits to improve insulin response

Sport and physical activity are meant to improve health and represent a valuable form of socialization and emotional well-being. Playing sports or simple daily exercises helps keep the body active, improving circulation, flexibility, and muscle strength. It also offers the opportunity to connect with other people and reduce stress. In a context where glucose management is essential, especially for those living with diabetes, regular physical activity contributes significantly to improving the insulin response.

Regular walks

Walking is one of the most accessible and beneficial forms of exercise for all ages. Even a daily 30-minute brisk walk can have surprising effects on health. This activity stimulates blood circulation, facilitating the transport of oxygen and nutrients to tissues, and increases fat oxidation, helping the body use glucose as an energy source more efficiently. Walking in the fresh air offers additional benefits: exposure to natural light helps regulate circadian rhythms, improving mood and sleep quality, while the ability to interact with others, perhaps during a group walk, adds a social aspect that contributes to overall emotional well-being.

Resistance Exercises

Resistance exercises, which include lightweight training or bodyweight exercises such as squats, push-ups, and sit-ups, are crucial for building muscle mass. Increased muscle mass improves daily strength and function. It is directly related to the body's improved ability to use glucose as fuel. This happens because muscles, being large energy consumers, require constant glucose availability and their increase promotes greater insulin sensitivity. In addition, these exercises contribute to a more efficient metabolism, helping to burn calories even at rest and maintain optimal body composition, which is crucial for managing blood sugar levels.

Yoga and Stretching

Yoga and stretching are complementary practices that go beyond just stretching muscles. These activities improve flexibility, strength, and balance, but they also play a crucial role in reducing stress. Yoga promotes greater awareness of the body and mind, lowering cortisol levels. This stress hormone in excess can negatively alter the insulin response and compromise metabolism. Stretching also helps improve circulation and prevent muscle tension, making the body more relaxed and ready to handle daily challenges. If integrated into a regular routine, these practices help stabilize blood sugar and improve overall psychophysical well-being.

Regular Meal and Night's Rest Schedules

Establishing a daily routine with fixed night rest times is key to optimizing metabolism and regulating blood sugar. Eating regularly helps the body synchronize digestive processes, ensuring constant and controlled assimilation of nutrients. This helps to avoid sudden swings in blood sugar levels, reducing the risk of blood sugar spikes and insulin resistance. At the same time, quality sleep is essential for the recovery and regulation of hormones, including insulin. Creating a nighttime routine, reducing distractions, and establishing a relaxing environment allows the body to rest properly, supporting the endocrine system and improving the insulin response throughout the day.

Detox techniques to reduce inflammation of the pancreas

The pancreas, located in the upper abdomen, plays a crucial role in regulating blood sugar levels and overall managing carbohydrate metabolism. In addition to producing insulin, the key hormone for allowing cells to absorb glucose, the pancreas also secretes other substances critical for digestion, such as pancreatic enzymes that help break down nutrients. However, when blood sugar levels remain consistently high due to unbalanced diets, sedentary lifestyles, or genetic predispositions, this gland can undergo chronic inflammation that progressively impairs its function.

Inflammation of the pancreas not only causes immediate problems, such as abdominal pain or alterations in digestion but can also promote the development of long-term metabolic dysfunctions, such as insulin resistance and type II diabetes. Suppose the pancreas can no longer produce insulin adequately, or the body's cells become less sensitive to this hormone. In that case, imbalances profoundly affect the quality of life. As a result, taking steps to reduce inflammation and protect the pancreas becomes essential to prevent metabolic complications, maintain reasonable glycemic control, and support long-lasting overall well-being.

When the pancreas is inflamed, its ability to produce insulin adequately can be impaired. If the amount of insulin secreted is insufficient, the glucose in the circulation struggles to enter the cells, leading to increased blood sugar levels. In addition, chronic inflammation can promote the appearance of insulin resistance, a phenomenon in which the body's cells no longer respond appropriately to insulin, further aggravating the problem. This condition forms the basis of numerous metabolic disorders, including type II diabetes. In addition to secreting insulin, the pancreas releases other hormones and enzymes that intervene in regulating carbohydrate metabolism. In persistent inflammation, these functions can be altered, leading to an imbalance in sugar management. Excess glucose, not being adequately absorbed by cells, tends to accumulate in the blood, causing hyperglycemia and, over time, favoring the onset of chronic diseases such as diabetes. A healthy pancreas, on the other hand, allows a correct metabolism of carbohydrates, ensuring a constant release of energy and preventing dangerous glycemic fluctuations. Chronic inflammation of the pancreas can trigger a broader inflammatory state involving the entire body. Free radicals and oxidative stress markers are generated when the body is constantly exposed to high sugar levels and prolonged metabolic stress. This condition, in turn, can further damage tissues and organs, including the liver and kidneys, establishing a vicious cycle of systemic inflammation. Reducing inflammation of the pancreas, therefore, helps improve insulin production but also helps limit the damage resulting from the continuous release of pro-inflammatory substances into the body.

Chronic inflammation can lead, in the long term, to structural damage to the cells of the pancreas, particularly those responsible for producing insulin (beta cells). When these cells are injured or die, the ability to regulate blood glucose levels is drastically reduced. In extreme cases, the damage can be so severe that it leads to pancreatic failure or forms of diabetes that are particularly difficult to manage. Acting promptly to reduce inflammation of the pancreas is crucial to maintain reasonable glycemic control and prevent metabolic complications that can compromise quality of life.

To support the function of the pancreas and promote cell regeneration, it is possible to adopt some specific detox techniques, which are integrated into an active lifestyle and an alkaline diet. Here are three key strategies:

Controlled intermittent fasting

Intermittent fasting is based on alternating eating periods with windows of time in which you avoid ingesting solid food. This practice, used in different cultural and religious traditions, has aroused the scientific community's interest in its possible benefits on metabolic health. During fasting, the body stops the constant production of insulin, allowing the pancreas to "recover" from the stress due to the continuous processing of sugars. Numerous studies have shown that intermittent fasting improves insulin sensitivity, promoting better blood sugar control and reducing the risk of developing insulin resistance. In addition, without a continuous influx of calories, the body tends to use fat stores more efficiently, helping to maintain a balanced weight. If applied gradually and controlled, this approach can reduce metabolic stress and facilitate cell regeneration, offering significant support to the pancreas and the entire digestive system.

Purifying herbal teas

Purifying herbal teas based on medicinal plants such as dandelion and milk thistle is a natural tool to promote detoxification and support the functionality of the liver, pancreas, and intestines. Dandelion is known for its diuretic action, which stimulates urine production and helps eliminate toxins accumulated in the body. This "cleansing" effect can relieve the load on the pancreas, allowing energy to be focused on producing and regulating digestive enzymes and insulin. On the other hand, milk thistle, thanks to its active ingredient called silymarin, has an antioxidant and regenerating action on liver cells. A liver in good condition, in fact, collaborates with the pancreas in the metabolism of nutrients and in the management of carbohydrates, helping to keep blood sugar levels stable. Regularly incorporating these herbal teas into your routine can reduce inflammatory processes, support hormonal balance, and improve overall well-being.

Constant hydration

Hydration is crucial in ensuring the proper functioning of all body systems, including the pancreatic system. Drinking water in adequate quantities, especially during fasting periods or between meals, supports the natural waste elimination processes, favoring the expulsion of toxins and waste substances. Maintaining a well-hydrated internal environment is essential for the pancreas, which can thus carry out its metabolic functions without excessive load. Adding a pinch of lemon or ginger to water can enhance the beneficial effect: lemon, rich in vitamin C and alkalizing substances, helps balance the body's pH, while ginger has anti-inflammatory properties that support digestive health. In the context of a balanced diet and regular physical activity, constant hydration is a fundamental element in improving the efficiency of the pancreas, reducing oxidative stress, and keeping the body in a state of lasting well-being.

A little reflection

The pancreas is a delicate organ, and, like many other health problems, we often look for immediate, fast, and undemanding solutions. However, in 90% of cases—except for diseases of genetic or hereditary origin—disorders and dysfunctions can be reduced or even eliminated thanks to a balanced diet and an adequate lifestyle.

Often, due to fatigue or stress related to work and other responsibilities, we rely on chemical drugs. Yet, these medicines contain substances found in nature in very high doses, capable of offering rapid relief but not always sustainable in the long term.

It is essential to consider staying healthy by focusing on a radical change in our relationship with food, exercise, and body care in general. Combined with a holistic and constant approach, natural remedies can make a difference and profoundly transform our lives, contributing to stable and lasting well-being.

Recommended and Avoiding Foods

Here is an example table, with 15 alkalizing foods or foods that are particularly beneficial for those who want to control glucose and support metabolism, alongside their main benefit:

Food	Benefit for Glucose Control and Metabolic Support
Spinach	Rich in magnesium and potassium, they help stabilize blood sugar levels and reduce inflammation.
Avocado	A source of healthy fats and fiber, it helps slow down the absorption of sugars and promotes satiety.
Quinoa	Non-hybridized whole grain, with a low glycemic impact, provides quality vegetable proteins and essential minerals.
Cucumbers	High in water and potassium, they help hydration and proper electrolyte balance, stabilizing blood sugar.
Ginger	It has anti-inflammatory properties and can improve insulin sensitivity, helping to control blood sugar spikes.
Almonds	Rich in unsaturated fats and vitamin E, they help keep blood sugar levels stable and provide constant energy.
Blueberries	High in antioxidants and fiber, it helps improve the insulin response and protect blood vessels.
Broccoli	Source of sulforaphane, a compound that supports liver detoxification and helps reduce inflammation.
Flaxseed	Rich in Omega-3 fatty acids and fiber, they help regulate blood sugar and promote cardiovascular health.
Whole barley	A cereal with a low glycemic index, it provides gradual energy and supports the intestinal bacterial flora.
Kale	High in vitamins and minerals, it contributes to pancreatic health and carbohydrate metabolism.
Tofu	Vegetable protein with a low glycemic index, it helps stabilize sugar levels and provide essential amino acids.
Carrots	Source of beta-carotene and fiber, they promote the regulation of sugar absorption and improve visual health.
Spelt (wholemeal)	Ancient cereal, more digestible than modern wheat, provides complex carbohydrates and useful micronutrients.
Aromatic herbs (rosemary, thyme)	In addition to flavoring dishes without resorting to salt, they contain antioxidant substances that support metabolism and circulation.

CHAPTER 10: DR SEBI AND HYPERTENSION

The Real Cause of High Blood Pressure According to Dr. Sebi

According to Dr. Sebi's approach, hypertension does not result only from an excess of salt or a simple hereditary factor but is rather the consequence of an unbalanced internal environment, characterized by an accumulation of metabolic waste and excessive acidity. Regular consumption of processed foods rich in saturated fats, refined sugars and chemical additives promotes the production of mucus and toxic residues, which are deposited on the walls of blood vessels, reducing their elasticity and hindering circulation. In addition, a body that is constantly in a state of acidity is more prone to chronic inflammation, a condition that exacerbates stress on the cardiovascular system and forces the heart to work harder to pump blood. Restoring a more alkaline pH through a diet based on natural and unprocessed foods, therefore, helps reduce the presence of metabolic waste, freeing blood vessels from unwanted accumulations and promoting a gradual return to normal blood pressure values.

Natural herbs to regulate blood pressure

1. Hawthorn (Crataegus monogyna)

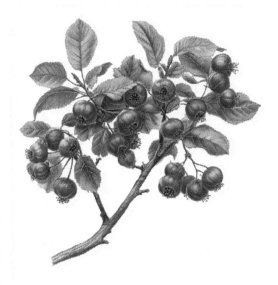

Hawthorn is widely recognized for its vasodilatory power and ability to improve blood circulation, which are key elements in managing high blood pressure. Its active ingredients, such as flavonoid and thymol, help relax the walls of blood vessels, reducing peripheral resistance and facilitating blood flow. This, in turn, allows the heart to pump with less effort and helps maintain a more balanced pressure.

Ingredients:

- 1 teaspoon dried hawthorn flowers
- 250 ml boiling water

Guidelines:

1. Bring the water to a boil.
2. Place the hawthorn flowers in a cup.
3. Pour boiling water over the flowers and cover the cup.
4. Leave to infuse for 10 minutes, then strain and drink hot.

Garlic (Allium sativum)

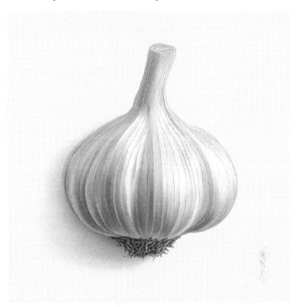

Garlic is a powerful natural ally in regulating blood pressure due to its ability to produce allicin, a compound that helps dilate blood vessels and reduce LDL cholesterol. These anti-inflammatory and antioxidant properties make garlic valuable for improving circulation and preventing plaque buildup, thereby reducing the risk of high blood pressure and cardiovascular complications.

Ingredients:

- 1 clove of fresh garlic
- 250 ml of water
- Juice of half a lemon

Guidelines:

1. Lightly crush the garlic clove to release its active compounds.
2. Put the garlic in a cup, add boiling water and lemon juice.
3. Leave to infuse for 5-7 minutes, then filter and consume warm.

Hibiscus (Hibiscus sabdariffa)

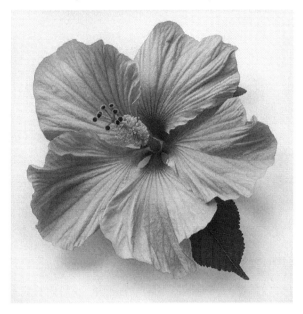

Hibiscus is known for its hypotensive and diuretic effect. Its properties, derived from anthocyanins and organic acids, promote the dilation of blood vessels and contribute to a reduction in water retention, two fundamental factors in keeping blood pressure under control. In addition, the acidic taste of hibiscus makes it a great base for refreshing and nourishing infusions.

Ingredients:

- 2 teaspoons dried hibiscus flowers
- 300 ml boiling water

Guidelines:
1. Place the hibiscus flowers in a teapot or cup.
2. Pour boiling water over the flowers.
3. Cover and leave to infuse for 10 minutes.
4. Filter and drink tea, hot or cold, depending on your preference.

Basil (Ocimum basilicum)

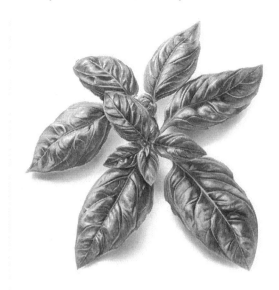

Basil, particularly in its aromatic varieties such as holy basil (Tulsi), contains eugenol and other compounds that promote vasodilation and reduce inflammation. These properties, combined with its calming effect on the nervous system, make basil useful for relieving tension that can contribute to hypertension.

Ingredients:

- 1 teaspoon fresh basil leaves
- 250 ml boiling water

Guidelines:
1. Wash the fresh basil leaves (if you use dried basil, proceed directly).
2. Place the basil in a cup and pour over the boiling water.
3. Cover and leave to infuse for 5-8 minutes.
4. Filter and consume the infusion to promote circulation and relaxation.

Dandelion (Taraxacum officinale)

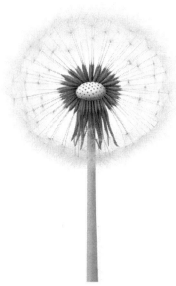

Dandelion is known for its diuretic and purifying properties. It stimulates the liver and kidneys, promoting the elimination of toxins that can stress the cardiovascular system. A purified and balanced body is less prone to developing hypertension problems.

Ingredients:

- 1 teaspoon dried dandelion root
- 250 ml boiling water
  Guidelines:
  1. Place the dandelion root in a cup.
  2. Pour boiling water over plant materials.
  3. Cover and leave to infuse for 10 minutes.
  4. Strain and consume the infusion, preferably in the morning to stimulate the detoxification system.

Passionflower (Passionflower incarnata)

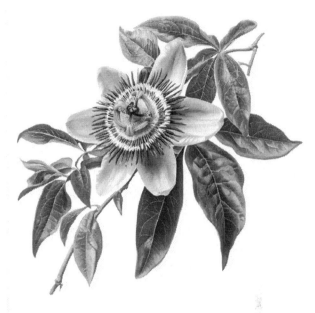

Passionflower is renowned for its anxiolytic and relaxing properties, which can help reduce stress – one of the main triggers of high blood pressure. It helps to improve sleep quality and calm the nervous system, reducing cortisol levels and thus promoting more stable blood pressure control.

Ingredients:

- 1 teaspoon dried passionflower leaves
- 250 ml boiling water
  Guidelines:
  1. Place the passionflower leaves in a cup.
  2. Pour boiling water over the leaves.
  3. Cover and leave to infuse for 5-7 minutes.
  4. Strain and drink the infusion, preferably in the evening, for a calming effect.

Orthosiphon (Orthosiphon stamineus)

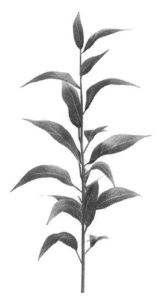

Orthosiphon is a plant of Asian origin with very marked diuretic properties, useful for reducing water retention and promoting the drainage of excess fluids. This diuretic effect helps to cleanse the system, improving kidney function and contributing to a more balanced blood pressure.

Ingredients:

- 1 teaspoon dried orthosiphon leaves
- 250 ml boiling water
  Guidelines:
  1. Place the leaves in a cup.
  2. Pour boiling water over the leaves.
  3. Cover and let steep for 7-10 minutes.
  4. Filter and consume the infusion to aid fluid drainage and purification.

Cardamom (Elettaria cardamomum)

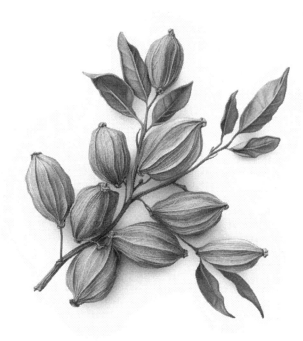

Cardamom is an aromatic spice rich in antioxidants, known for its slightly vasodilator and diuretic effect. It promotes better circulation and helps counteract fluid accumulation, thanks to its ability to stimulate metabolism and improve digestion.

Ingredients:

- 2-3 crushed cardamom berries
- 250 ml boiling water
  Guidelines:
  1. Lightly crush the cardamom berries to release their essential oils.
  2. Put the berries in a cup and pour boiling water over them.
  3. Cover and leave to infuse for 5-8 minutes.
  4. Filter and drink the tea, ideal for stimulating digestion and circulation.

These natural remedies, prepared with simple infusions and decoctions, offer a practical way to integrate the beneficial properties of herbs into everyday life. Using these combinations on a regular basis can help support the immune system and promote overall well-being, helping to keep blood pressure in balance and protecting heart health.

The Role of Sodium and Potassium in the Alkaline Diet

The correct balance of sodium and potassium is essential for maintaining stable blood pressure and for the health of the cardiovascular system. These two minerals work synergistically to regulate the body's fluid balance, directly influencing water retention and plasma volume and determining blood pressure. Excess sodium, typically associated with diets high in processed foods and added salts, can lead to water retention and increased blood pressure. At the same time, adequate potassium intake helps dilate blood vessels, facilitate blood flow, and reduce blood pressure spikes.

Several scientific studies have shown that a diet rich in potassium – abundant in fruits and vegetables – can help reduce the risk of hypertension. For example, research published in the *Journal of the American College of Cardiology* has shown that a high potassium/sodium ratio is associated with a lower incidence of cardiovascular disease. Similarly, an article in *Hypertension Research* emphasized the importance of limiting sodium intake to prevent hydro electrolyte stress and increased blood pressure, highlighting that an alkaline diet, naturally low in sodium and high in potassium, offers a more balanced internal environment.

Potassium's vasodilator effect helps reduce blood pressure. It is also essential for the proper functioning of muscle and nerve cells, contributing to effective heart contraction and better communication between tissues. Adequate potassium intake also promotes the elimination of excess fluids, thus preventing cardiovascular system overload and reducing the risk of edema.

A correct balance between sodium and potassium is a pillar of the alkaline diet, as it allows you to limit water retention and maintain a balanced blood pressure. Adopting a diet that promotes potassium intake – through the consumption of fruits, vegetables, and legumes – and that reduces foods with a high sodium content represents a scientifically supported strategy to protect the heart and improve overall health.

Strategies to reduce stress and improve circulation

Chronic stress is one of the main contributing factors to cardiovascular health, as it causes an increase in the production of cortisol and other stress hormones, which can force blood vessels to constrict and suffer damage over time. Constant tension generates a state of hypervigilance that increases blood pressure and promotes the onset of systemic inflammation, making the circulatory system more vulnerable to diseases such as hypertension and atherosclerosis. On the other hand, optimal blood circulation is essential for the well-being of the body, as it ensures the effective transport of oxygen and nutrients to all tissues and facilitates the elimination of toxins. For this reason, reducing stress and adopting a regular physical activity routine are complementary and indispensable strategies to lighten the load on blood vessels and promote overall well-being.

Relaxation techniques, such as meditation, deep breathing, and mindfulness, help reduce cortisol levels and restore a hormonal balance conducive to blood vessel dilation. At the same time, moderate physical activities – such as walking, yoga, tai chi, and stretching – stimulate blood flow, strengthen muscles, and improve artery flexibility, making the cardiovascular system more efficient. These practices reduce mental stress and promote circulation, contributing to better oxygenation of tissues and a more extraordinary ability of the body to regenerate. In this way, the combination of stress management and physical movement becomes a powerful ally in the prevention of cardiovascular disease and in maintaining optimal health.

"Breathe & Walk" routine:

Step 1: Start your day by dedicating 5 minutes to meditation or deep breathing. Find a quiet place to sit comfortably, close your eyes, and focus your attention on your breathing. Inhale slowly through your nose, holding your breath for a few seconds, then slowly exhale through your mouth. This simple exercise helps calm the mind, lower cortisol levels, and prepare the body for a day of movement, reducing anxiety and promoting mental clarity.

Step 2: Continue with a 20–30-minute walk at a brisk pace, preferably in the fresh air. Choose a pleasant route, perhaps in a park or along a path, where you can enjoy natural light and contact with nature. Walking steadily stimulates blood circulation, promotes tissue oxygenation, and activates the muscular system, helping to reduce stress and improve cardiovascular health.

Step 3: During the walk, focus your attention on your breathing and body movement, practicing mindfulness. Try to perceive every step, the rhythm of your breathing, the sound of your steps on the surface, and the air around you. This approach helps you reduce psychological stress, improve concentration, and transform walking into a moment of active meditation, were mind and body work in synergy.

Step 4: At the end of the walk, dedicate yourself to stretching exercises. Focus on stretching the muscles in your legs, back, and arms, performing slow, controlled movements. Stretching promotes muscle relaxation and helps dilate blood vessels, further improving circulation and preventing muscle stiffness. Spend 5-10 minutes on this phase, focusing on breathing to maximize the relaxing effect.

Step 5: Integrate this routine into your daily routine, practicing it at least 3-4 times weekly. Consistent exercise improves cardiovascular health and circulation and contributes to long-lasting mental well-being, reducing stress levels and promoting optimal mental and physical balance. Over time, this routine will become an essential part of your lifestyle, helping you maintain energy, clarity, and serenity daily.

Foods to avoid at all costs for those suffering from hypertension

For those living with hypertension, adopting a balanced, alkaline diet is crucial to keep blood pressure under control and prevent long-term complications. According to Dr. Sebi's approach and modern nutritional evidence, certain foods can increase systemic inflammation, promote water retention, and excessively stress the cardiovascular system. These foods, typically rich in sodium, refined sugars, and saturated fats, act synergistically to cause an imbalance in pH and an increase in oxidative stress levels, elements that contribute significantly to the rise in blood pressure. Avoiding or minimizing these foods allows you to relieve the load on blood vessels, promote better circulation, and promote a more alkaline internal environment, which is essential for heart health. Below is a detailed list of foods and ingredients to be restricted, with concrete examples of which foods are found:

Table salt and foods high in sodium

Why avoid: Excess sodium causes the body to retain fluids, increasing blood volume and blood pressure.

Where to find it: Table salt, salty snacks (chips, crackers), canned foods, ready-to-eat soups, industrial condiments and sauces, smoked foods, and sausages.

Refined sugars and industrial sweets

Why avoid: Refined sugars cause blood sugar spikes and promote inflammation, contributing to metabolic stress and acid waste formation.

Where to find it: White sugar, high-fructose corn syrup, packaged sweets, cookies, cakes, industrial chocolate, sugary drinks, and fruit juices with added sugars.

Saturated fats and fried foods

Why avoid: Excessive intake of saturated fat contributes to increased LDL cholesterol ("bad" cholesterol) and plaque formation in the arteries, aggravating high blood pressure.

Where to find it: Fatty red meats, aged cheeses, full-fat dairy products, butter, palm oil, fried foods (French fries, croquettes, fried snacks), and fast food.

Processed and industrial foods

Why avoid: Highly processed foods contain numerous additives, preservatives, and often high amounts of sodium and sugar, which increase inflammation and contribute to an acidic environment in the body.

Where to find it: Ready meals, frozen meals, packaged foods, sausages, sausages, industrial snacks and pre-packaged foods.

Alcoholic beverages

Why avoid: Alcohol can increase blood pressure, promote dehydration, and contribute to chronic inflammation by interfering with metabolic balance.

Where to find it: Wine, beer, hard liquor, and cocktails, especially those containing added sugar.

Commercial bakery products

Why avoid: They often contain high amounts of sugar, trans fats, and salt, contributing to inflammation and increased blood pressure.

Where to find it: Industrial bread, biscuits, packaged sweets, croissants, and other baked goods.

Industrial condiments and sauces

Why avoid: These products contain high sodium, sugars, and additives, which can alter electrolyte balance and increase water retention.

Where to find it: Ketchup, industrial mayonnaise, pasta, salad dressings, and soy-based sauces.

Reducing the consumption of these foods is essential for those suffering from hypertension. Limiting salt and sugar intake and preferring fresh, whole, and naturally alkaline foods helps maintain water balance and reduce systemic inflammation. In addition, eliminating or minimizing processed foods helps protect the cardiovascular system, improves circulation, and supports more stable blood pressure over time.

Adopting these dietary strategies is essential in reducing the risk of complications associated with high blood pressure and promoting long-term heart health.

Infusions and herbal teas for a healthy heart

Infusions and herbal teas are a simple, natural, and highly effective method to support heart and muscle health. These drinks, prepared with medicinal herbs, offer many benefits thanks to their antioxidant, anti-inflammatory, and vasodilator properties. Herbal drinks help relax muscles and blood vessels, promoting better circulation and reducing the workload on the heart. In addition, the antioxidants present in many herbal teas counteract oxidative stress. This key factor contributes to the premature aging of cardiovascular cells. The relaxation induced by these infusions can reduce cortisol levels, improving overall well-being and contributing to quality sleep, which is essential for cell regeneration. In addition, some infusions promote detoxification of the body, helping the liver eliminate toxins and thus maintain a more balanced internal environment that is less prone to inflammation.

Hawthorn herbal tea

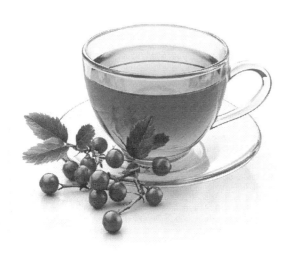

Prep Time: 5 min,
Ingredients:

- 1 teaspoon dried hawthorn flowers
- 250 ml boiling water

Instructions:

1. Bring the water to a boil.
2. Place the hawthorn flowers in a cup.
3. Pour boiling water over the flowers and cover the cup.
4. Leave to infuse for 10 minutes, then filter.
5. Drink the hot tea. This herbal tea promotes the dilation of blood vessels and improves circulation, helping to reduce blood pressure and support heart health. In addition, the anti-inflammatory properties of the compounds found in hawthorn help strengthen the immune system.

Hibiscus herbal tea

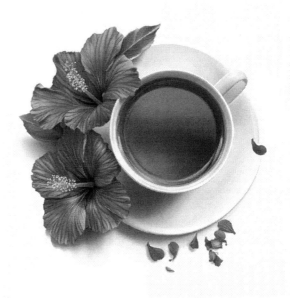

Preparation time: 5 min, Infusion: 10 min,
Ingredients:

- 2 teaspoons dried hibiscus flowers
- 300 ml boiling water

Instructions:

1. Bring the water to a boil.
2. Place the hibiscus flowers in a teapot or cup.
3. Pour boiling water over the flowers.
4. Cover and leave to infuse for 10 minutes.
5. Strain the brew and drink hot or cold. Hibiscus is known for its diuretic and hypotensive effect; It helps reduce water retention and dilate blood vessels, promoting better circulation and counteracting oxidative stress thanks to anthocyanins.

Thyme infusion

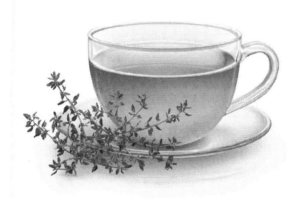

Preparation time: 5 min, Infusion: 7 min,
Ingredients:

- 1 teaspoon dried thyme leaves
- 250 ml boiling water

    Instructions:
1. Bring the water to a boil.
2. Place the thyme in a cup.
3. Pour boiling water over the thyme flowers.
4. Cover and leave to infuse for 7 minutes.
5. Strain and drink the hot infusion.

Thyme has antiseptic and vasodilator properties, which help improve blood circulation and relax the cardiovascular system. Its calming effect also supports respiratory function and general well-being.

Dandelion Herbal Tea

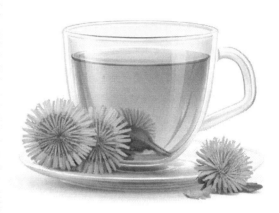

Preparation time: 5 min, Infusion: 10 min,
Ingredients:

- 1 teaspoon dried dandelion root
- 250 ml boiling water

    Instructions:
1. Bring the water to a boil.
2. Place the dandelion root in a cup.
3. Pour boiling water over plant materials.
4. Cover and leave to infuse for 10 minutes.
5. Filter the infusion and drink hot, preferably in the morning to stimulate the purification system.

Dandelion promotes diuresis and purification, helping the liver and kidneys to eliminate toxins. This supports the cardiovascular system by reducing excess fluid load and keeping pressure in balance.

Rosemary infusion

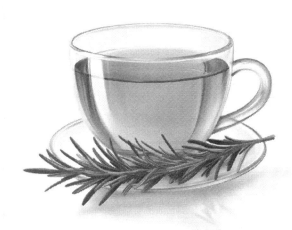

Preparation time: 5 min, Infusion: 7-10 min,
Ingredients:

- 1 teaspoon dried rosemary leaves
- 250 ml boiling water

Instructions:
1. Bring the water to a boil.
2. Place the rosemary in a cup.
3. Pour boiling water over the rosemary flowers.
4. Cover and let steep for 7-10 minutes.
5. Strain and drink the hot infusion.

Rosemary stimulates circulation and has anti-inflammatory and antioxidant properties that protect the heart and muscle cells. It is also known to improve concentration and support memory, contributing to overall well-being.

Passionflower Herbal Tea

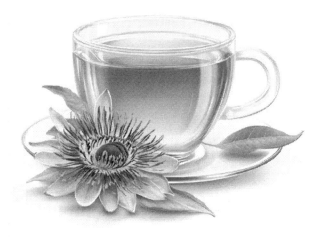

Prep Time: 5 min, Infusion: 5-7 min,
Ingredients

- 1 teaspoon dried passionflower leaves
- 250 ml boiling water

Instructions:
1. Bring the water to a boil.
2. Place the passionflower leaves in a cup.
3. Pour boiling water over the leaves.
4. Cover and leave to infuse for 5-7 minutes.
5. Filter and drink the hot infusion, preferably in the evening to promote relaxation. Passionflower helps reduce stress and anxiety, promoting a calming effect on the nervous system. These relaxing benefits can help stabilize blood pressure, especially at times when stress plays a major role.

Chamomile and Ginger infusion

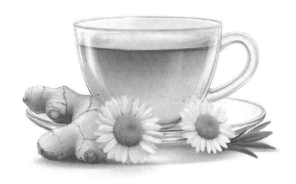

Preparation time: 5 min, Infusion: 5-7 min,
Ingredients:

- 1 teaspoon of chamomile flowers
- 3-4 slices of fresh ginger
- 250 ml boiling water

Instructions:

1. Bring the water to a boil.
2. Put the chamomile flowers and ginger in a cup.
3. Pour boiling water over the ingredients.
4. Cover and leave to infuse for 5-7 minutes.
5. Strain and drink the hot infusion. This infusion combines the soothing and calming properties of chamomile with the anti-inflammatory and digestive abilities of ginger. The result is a remedy that promotes relaxation, improves digestion and supports circulation, contributing to cardiovascular health in a natural way.

Catechins

Catechins are antioxidant compounds found in abundance in green tea and are one of the main reasons why this drink is considered an ally in the fight against body fat. Catechins, epigallocatechin gallate (EGCG), play a key role in increasing lipid metabolism: they help stimulate thermogenesis, i.e. the process in which the body burns calories to produce heat, and facilitate the oxidation of fats, making it more efficient to use fat reserves as a source of energy.

An important aspect is when you take green tea to maximize its benefits. It is generally recommended to drink it between meals, preferably during the postprandial phase (i.e. a few hours after eating) or at times when the stomach is relatively empty. This is because, during meals, the presence of food can interfere with the absorption and effectiveness of catechins. When the body is not engaged in the digestion of nutrients, catechins can act more freely, helping to stimulate metabolism and promote fat burning. Drinking green tea between meals helps to avoid possible interference between the compounds present in food and catechins, ensuring that the latter can be optimally absorbed. In this way, the thermogenic potential of green tea is fully exploited, which, together with its antioxidant effect, protects cells from free radical damage and supports a healthy metabolism.

Green tea catechins are a powerful natural tool for improving fat burning and promoting weight loss. Taking them between meals allows you to maximize their effect, as the body, not engaged in digestion, can more effectively use these substances to speed up metabolism and transform fat into energy, helping to maintain a healthier and fitter body.

CHAPTER 11: AUTOIMMUNE DISEASES

Autoimmune diseases represent a set of conditions in which the immune system, instead of protecting the body, mistakenly attacks healthy tissues. This phenomenon, which can occur in numerous organs and systems, is often the result of chronic inflammation and internal imbalances involving the intestine, mucus, and the entire cellular environment. Chronic inflammation, in fact, is not simply a temporary response to an infection or trauma but becomes a persistent state that progressively damages cells and tissues, predisposing the body to autoimmune reactions. This continuous inflammatory condition is closely related to an imbalanced intestine: a compromised intestinal barrier, together with an altered bacterial flora, allows the passage of undigested substances, toxins, and antigens into the bloodstream, triggering an incorrect immune response that results in the attack of healthy tissues.

According to some natural approaches, such as the one proposed by Dr. Sebi, the key to preventing and managing autoimmune diseases lies in restoring internal balance through a diet based on alkaline principles. Dr. Sebi's philosophy holds that many chronic diseases originate from an excessively acidic body environment, which favors the accumulation of metabolic waste and persistent inflammation. This imbalance damages cells and compromises the function of the intestine, creating a condition favorable to the development of autoimmune reactions.

Adopting an alkaline diet means favoring natural, whole, plant-based foods, which help maintain a balanced pH in the body and reduce systemic inflammation. In addition to this, the use of specific herbs, detox techniques, and stress management practices are configured as complementary strategies to rebalance the immune system. Dr. Sebi proposes, in fact, a holistic approach that does not limit itself to treating the symptoms but aims to intervene in the root causes: by eliminating processed foods rich in refined sugars and chemicals and replacing them with fresh and alkalizing foods, it is possible to promote lasting cell regeneration and restoration of the well-being of the entire body.

This philosophy, which integrates nutrition, herbs, and an active lifestyle, offers a long-lasting remedy for autoimmune problems. Following Dr. Sebi's principles, the body is gradually cleansed of toxins, chronic inflammation is reduced, and the intestine, the heart of immune health, is restored to an optimal state. The result is a decrease in autoimmune crises, an improvement in quality of life, and a more extraordinary ability of the body to self-regulate and defend itself naturally.

The role of inflammation in autoimmune diseases

Chronic inflammation is a prolonged state of activation of the immune system that, instead of resolving an infection or repairing damage, persists and feeds itself over time. This phenomenon can occur due to several factors, including an excessively acidifying diet, the constant presence of environmental toxins, and chronic stress, which alter the body's pH balance and create an environment conducive to prolonged inflammatory processes. When subjected to persistent inflammation, immune cells, such as T lymphocytes and macrophages, are activated continuously. In this context, they may begin to mistakenly recognize healthy tissues as threats, triggering an autoimmune response that leads to progressive damage to organs and systems.

The mechanism behind this phenomenon is complex: an acidic environment due to a diet rich in refined sugars, industrial foods, and saturated fats generates toxins and metabolic waste that persist in the body. These substances, in turn, stimulate an inflammatory response that never resolves completely. Immune cells, constantly on alert, end up attacking even healthy tissues, upsetting the balance of the body and causing damage that accumulates over time. Chronic inflammation, therefore, acts like a seed from which numerous autoimmune diseases are born, such as multiple sclerosis, rheumatoid arthritis, systemic lupus erythematosus, and many other debilitating conditions.

Reducing inflammation through correct food choices, using natural remedies, and eliminating toxins are essential to breaking this vicious cycle. Adopting a diet based on whole and alkaline foods, for example, can help restore the balance of internal pH, thus reducing the production of acidifying waste and limiting the excessive activation of the immune system. In this way, the body can regenerate cells and restore optimal functioning, preventing the progress of autoimmune diseases and relieving related symptoms.

The connection between mucus, gut, and autoimmune diseases

Intestinal mucus protects the digestive tract as a barrier against pathogens, toxins, and undigested food particles. However, excess mucus or its altered composition can indicate an intestinal imbalance, significantly affecting the immune system. When the intestine is inflamed or the mucous barrier is compromised – a phenomenon known as "leaky gut" or increased intestinal permeability – substances usually contained in the intestinal lumen can enter the bloodstream. This translocation of antigens and toxins activates an abnormal immune response, as the immune system, unexpectedly exposed to these "intruders," can begin to recognize the body's own tissues as foreign ones, contributing to the development of autoimmune diseases.

In addition, a poorly maintained intestine, characterized by an unbalanced bacterial flora (dysbiosis), promotes excess mucus production. Such abnormal mucus production is often the result of chronic inflammation, which, in turn, can further worsen intestinal permeability. This vicious cycle of inflammation, dysbiosis, and increased mucus production impairs the body's ability to maintain a balanced immune system and can trigger autoimmune reactions. Gut well-being is, therefore, closely linked to the health of the immune system, and the regulation of mucus production through a balanced diet and the use of probiotics and natural remedies can help prevent or mitigate autoimmune diseases.

Leaky Gut

Leaky gut, often called "leaky gut," is a condition in which the typically highly selective and protective intestinal barrier loses its ability to retain toxins, bacteria, and undigested food particles. In a healthy gut, epithelial cells form a barrier supplemented by tight junctions that prevent the indiscriminate passage of substances from the intestinal lumen into the bloodstream. However, factors such as a diet rich in processed foods and refined sugars, excessive antibiotic intake, chronic stress, and other metabolic dysfunctions can weaken these junctions, making the barrier too permeable.

When this imbalance occurs, particles and toxins that would usually be eliminated are translocated into the bloodstream, triggering an abnormal immune response. The immune system, which is constantly activated by these intruders, produces chronic inflammation, which in turn contributes to further damage to intestinal mucosa cells. This vicious cycle of persistent inflammation not only impairs the digestive tract's efficiency but can also trigger autoimmune reactions, in which the body begins to attack its own tissues, mistakenly perceiving them as threats.

Microbiota, Prebiotics and Probiotics

The gut microbiota, the collection of bacteria, viruses, and other microorganisms that inhabit our gut, plays a crucial role in regulating the immune system and maintaining overall health. A balanced intestinal flora is essential to keep the mucosal barrier in good health, as it controls mucus production, preventing excesses that could promote more excellent intestinal permeability and the onset of the so-called "leaky gut." These microorganisms, in fact, constantly interact with the immune system, educating it to distinguish between harmless substances and potential threats and helping to modulate the inflammatory response to prevent autoimmune reactions. The integration of probiotics and prebiotics into the diet is crucial to strengthen this ecosystem: probiotics, which are live microorganisms found in fermented foods such as yogurt, kefir, sauerkraut, and kimchi, help maintain an optimal composition of the intestinal flora, while prebiotics – dietary fibers that act as "food" for beneficial bacteria – are found in foods such as garlic, onion, bananas, asparagus, and chicory root. These essential nutrients help prevent dysbiosis, strengthening the gut barrier and reducing the risk of systemic inflammation and autoimmune conditions. This integrated approach aligns perfectly with Dr. Sebi's philosophy, who argued that a balanced, alkaline indoor environment, achieved through natural nutrition and herbal remedies, is crucial for overall well-being. According to Dr. Sebi, maintaining a healthy gut microbiota is one of the keys to promoting cell regeneration, reducing inflammation, and preventing many chronic diseases afflicting humans. Supplementing probiotics and prebiotics improves gut health and contributes to a stronger immune system and better energy management, creating a virtuous circle that supports long-term health and reflects the principles of balance and harmony promoted by its philosophy.

Natural remedies

Restoring the intestinal mucosal barrier is critical to overall health, as it is the first line of defense against toxins, bacteria, and other potentially harmful substances entering the bloodstream. When the mucosal barrier is compromised, the so-called "leaky gut" condition occurs, which allows antigens and toxins to pass into the bloodstream, triggering inappropriate immune responses and chronic inflammation. For this reason, restoring and maintaining a healthy gut barrier is essential for preventing autoimmune disorders and other chronic diseases.

Numerous natural remedies can support this regenerative process. Certain nutrients and herbs, such as glutamine, are crucial for regenerating the epithelial cells that make up the intestinal mucosa, repairing cracks, and strengthening the barrier. Other plants, such as dandelion and milk thistle, play a purifying role, helping to reduce inflammation and promote the elimination of toxins, thus creating an internal environment more favorable to cell regeneration. In addition, foods rich in omega-3s, antioxidants, and essential vitamins provide the necessary nutrients to support the intestinal mucosa's health and maintain a balanced immune system.

Below is a detailed list of the leading natural remedies for restoring and maintaining the mucosal barrier:

Glutamine

Glutamine is an amino acid essential for the regeneration of epithelial cells in the intestine. It helps repair cracks in the intestinal mucosa, improving the barrier that prevents toxins from entering. Glutamine can be taken through supplements or foods such as bone broth, lean meat, or certain plant products.

Dandelion

Dandelion is a purifying plant highly prized for its diuretic and detoxifying properties. It promotes the elimination of toxins, supporting liver and kidney function, and helps reduce intestinal inflammation. It can be taken in the form of herbal teas, decoctions, or extracts.

Milk thistle

Milk thistle is a medicinal herb rich in silymarin, a powerful antioxidant that can protect and regenerate liver cells. This liver-supporting action positively impacts gut health, helping to reduce inflammation. It is usually used in herbal teas, powders, or capsules.

Omega-3

Omega-3s are essential fatty acids with potent anti-inflammatory properties. They help reduce systemic inflammation and support cell membrane health, including intestinal mucosa. Omega-3s are found in flaxseed, chia seeds, walnuts, and fatty fish (such as salmon and mackerel). They can also be taken through fish oil supplements.

Turmeric

Turmeric is a spice known for its powerful anti-inflammatory and antioxidant effects, mainly due to curcumin. It can reduce inflammation in the gut and protect epithelial cells from oxidative stress. Turmeric can be added to foods, used in herbal teas, or taken as a powdered supplement.

Ginger

Ginger is a root with a characteristic warming and anti-inflammatory effect. It supports digestion, helps reduce inflammation, and stimulates circulation, helping to maintain a healthy intestinal barrier. It can be eaten fresh, in herbal teas, or as a condiment in recipes.

Probiotics

Probiotics are beneficial microorganisms that support the health of the gut microbiota. They promote the balance of bacterial flora, strengthening the intestinal barrier and lowering the risk of inflammation and excessive permeability. They are found in foods such as natural yogurt, kefir, sauerkraut, and kimchi or in probiotic blends and specific supplements.

Prebiotics

Prebiotics are dietary fibers that act as "food" for probiotics, stimulating the growth of beneficial bacteria and contributing to a balanced microbiota and a more robust gut barrier. They are in garlic, onion, bananas, asparagus, chicory root, and other inulin-rich foods.

Vitamin A

Vitamin A is essential for cell regeneration and supports the health of the intestinal mucosa. It helps maintain an integrated cell barrier and offers protection against infection. It is present in carrots, sweet potatoes, spinach, and cabbage and can also be taken in supplement form.

Vitamin C

Vitamin C is a powerful antioxidant that protects cells from oxidative stress. It strengthens the immune system, helps maintain mucosal health, and promotes cell regeneration. It is found in citrus fruits, strawberries, kiwis, peppers, and leafy greens.

Vitamin E

Vitamin E, known for its antioxidant effect, supports the health of cell membranes. It protects intestinal cells from oxidative damage and helps maintain the integrity of the mucosal barrier. It is in nuts, seeds, vegetable oils, and leafy greens.

These natural remedies, when integrated into a balanced diet and an active lifestyle, offer essential support for restoring and maintaining the intestinal mucosal barrier. These foods and supplements can help prevent toxins from entering, reduce inflammation, and improve immune system functioning, thus creating a solid foundation for long-term well-being.

Herbs and natural remedies to rebalance the immune system

A strong and well-functioning immune system is the key to defending against infections and diseases and maintaining optimal well-being in the long term. A balanced immune system helps fight pathogens and inflammation. It is crucial for ensuring consistent energy, good digestion, and overall health, allowing you to live fit and with vitality. In an era in which stress, pollution, and poor eating habits are commonplace, strengthening the immune system becomes essential to prevent numerous diseases and improve the quality of daily life.

Natural remedies and medicinal herbs represent a valid alternative to the classic chemical treatments often prescribed by modern medicine. While synthetic medications usually offer immediate relief, they can have long-term side effects and sometimes do not address the root causes of immune imbalance. Several scientific studies support the use of natural remedies: a study published in the *Journal of Ethnopharmacology* highlighted how many traditional herbs can modulate the immune response in a more balanced and sustainable way than synthetic drugs; an article in the *Journal of Alternative and Complementary Medicine* highlighted the benefits of plant extracts in reducing chronic inflammation. At the same time, phytotherapy research has shown that regular use of adaptogenic herbs can help reduce cortisol levels and improve stress resilience, key factors for an effective immune system. These studies indicate that the natural approach, based on the use of herbs and nutrients from nature, is not only in line with ancient wisdom but is also supported by modern scientific evidence that attests to its effectiveness in promoting a lasting immune balance.

Echinacea

Echinacea is renowned for stimulating the production of white blood cells, strengthening the body's defenses against viruses and bacteria. Its benefits are particularly evident during periods when the immune system is most stressed, such as the cold or flu season. It is instrumental in autumn and winter, when respiratory infections are more prevalent. Echinacea is commonly used in the form of herbal teas, tinctures, and supplements, but it can also be found in commercial preparations dedicated to immune support.

Astragalus

Rich in immunomodulating polysaccharides, astragalus is a powerful immune system booster, particularly indicated during stress and fatigue. This traditional remedy, widely used in Chinese medicine, is excellent for winter when the body needs more support to fight seasonal diseases. Astragalus usually comes as a dried root, which can be prepared in decoctions or herbal teas and integrated into capsules.

Ashwagandha (Withania somnifera)

Ashwagandha is one of the most popular adaptogenic herbs. It helps regulate cortisol levels and improve the immune response, promoting mental and physical balance. Thanks to its anti-stress properties, it is ideal during increased emotional pressure or intense work. It is recommended all year round, but especially in times of chronic stress. It can be taken as a powder to be mixed into drinks or capsules and is widely used in Ayurvedic medicine.

Elderberry (flowers and berries)

Elderberry possesses powerful antiviral and antioxidant properties, making it an excellent remedy for seasonal infections and strengthening the defenses of the respiratory tract. It is advantageous in spring and autumn when the changes of seasons favor the occurrence of colds and flu. Elderberry can be consumed as herbal teas, syrups, or supplements and is readily available as a preparation in pharmacies or herbalist's shops.

Reishi (Ganoderma lucidum)

Reishi is a medicinal mushroom known to modulate the immune response and reduce systemic inflammation. Thanks to its adaptogenic properties, it helps strengthen the body's defenses, which is useful in periods of chronic stress and during the winter seasons, when the immune system is most stressed. Reishi is usually consumed in powder, capsules, or liquid extracts and is often used in combination with other herbs for a synergistic effect.

Tulsi (Holy Basil)

Tulsi, or holy basil, is known for its adaptogenic and stress-relieving properties, making it an excellent ally for boosting the immune system. It helps reduce cortisol levels, improve emotional balance, and support against infections. It is especially recommended when stress and infections increase during seasonal transition periods, such as spring and autumn. Tulsi can be used in herbal teas, infusions, and decoctions and is often grown fresh in gardens.

Turmeric

Thanks to curcumin, turmeric offers powerful anti-inflammatory and antioxidant effects, protecting cells from free radical damage and modulating the immune response. It is ideal to use during chronic inflammation or when the immune system needs extra support, such as during winter. Turmeric is versatile and can be added to dishes, smoothies, herbal teas, or as a powdered supplement. It is often used in cooking in Indian and Asian traditions.

Ginger

Ginger is prized for its anti-inflammatory and digestive properties. It improves circulation and transports essential nutrients to the immune system. It helps soothe inflammation and supports digestion, making it an ideal remedy during colder and chilly times. Ginger is readily available fresh, dried, or powdered and can be used to prepare herbal teas, decoctions, or as a condiment in recipes.

Olives and extra virgin olive oil

Olives and extra virgin olive oil are rich in antioxidants and healthy fats, essential in controlling inflammation and supporting immune function. These foods are crucial for the Mediterranean diet, which is known for its cardiovascular benefits and the promotion of a controlled inflammatory state. Olives can be eaten as snacks or added to salads, while extra virgin olive oil is ideal for seasoning dishes and cooking at low temperatures, preserving their beneficial properties.

Aloe Vera

Aloe vera promotes cell regeneration and soothes inflammation, improving nutrient absorption and gut health, a key element for a balanced immune system. Its regenerating properties make it particularly useful in times of stress or during recovery phases, and it is recommended especially in spring and autumn. Aloe vera can be taken in the form of juice, gels, or supplements and is often used to cleanse and calm the digestive tract.

Vitamin C (from natural sources)

Vitamin C is a powerful antioxidant essential for the proper functioning of the immune system. It promotes tissue regeneration, protects cells from oxidative stress, and improves the ability to fight infections. It is beneficial during winter when respiratory infections are more common but valid all year round. Natural sources of vitamin C include citrus fruits, strawberries, kiwis, peppers, and leafy greens, which can be eaten fresh or used to make juices and smoothies.

Prebiotics and Probiotics

Prebiotics and probiotics are two fundamental pillars for intestinal health and, by extension, for the body's general well-being. Prebiotics are non-digestible dietary fibers that act as "food" for the beneficial bacteria in our gut, stimulating their growth and activity. These fibers reach the large intestine intact, where they are fermented by microorganisms, helping to create a favorable environment for producing short-chain fatty acids, such as butyrate, which play a key role in protecting the intestinal barrier and modulating the immune response.

On the other hand, probiotics are live microorganisms that, when taken in adequate amounts, help maintain or restore a healthy gut flora balance. These beneficial bacteria counteract the presence of pathogenic organisms, improve digestion, promote nutrient absorption, and help strengthen the immune system. A balanced microbiota not only supports gut health but also influences numerous aspects of overall well-being, including mood and metabolic function.

Foods rich in prebiotics support beneficial bacterial flora and improve gut health and overall well-being. Garlic and onion, for example, contain inulin and fructans that stimulate the growth of bacteria, which is helpful for digestion, making dishes tastier and, at the same time, friendly to the intestine. Bananas, especially those not yet fully ripe, also stand out for their contribution of prebiotic fibers that promote the expansion of healthy intestinal flora: an ideal addition for smoothies or quick and nutritious snacks.

Asparagus, known for its richness in inulin, supports intestinal fermentation and helps keep the mucosa in good condition. This vegetable, appreciated by those looking to vary their diet with light and tasty dishes, can be steamed, sautéed, or used as a base for spring soups. On the other hand, Chicory root is one of the most concentrated sources of inulin, essential for nourishing probiotics and improving intestinal function. It benefits those who want a barley or chicory coffee without sacrificing taste but limiting caffeine intake. Legumes, such as beans, lentils, and chickpeas, offer a valuable supply of prebiotic fibers capable of regulating intestinal transit and preventing dysbiosis. For those in charge of feeding an entire family, it is possible to offer these foods in soups, soups, or cold salads, varying the recipes according to preferences and seasons. Finally, green leafy fruits and vegetables represent a pillar of any wellness-oriented diet: their combination of soluble and insoluble fibers strengthens the intestinal barrier and encourages the growth of beneficial bacteria, contributing to a stable balance of the microbiota. Those who try to maintain an alkaline diet will find these vegetables fundamental to the entire body's health.

By integrating these foods into your daily diet, you can significantly improve the balance of your intestinal flora. The correct intake of prebiotics, combined with the consumption of probiotics through fermented foods such as yogurt, kefir, sauerkraut, and kimchi, creates an internal environment that promotes better digestion, more excellent protection against pathogens, and a strengthening of the immune system. This synergy is significant for preventing the onset of chronic diseases and for maintaining a healthy gut and a robust mucosal barrier.

Therefore, adopting a diet that includes prebiotics and probiotics is a fundamental step in improving intestinal health and positively affecting immune function and overall well-being. Numerous scientific studies published in journals such as the *Journal of Nutrition* and the *British Journal of Nutrition*, confirm that a diet rich in these components can reduce intestinal inflammation, improve digestion, and contribute to optimal metabolic balance. In summary, combining prebiotics and probiotics represents a natural and sustainable approach to keeping our intestines in perfect harmony, thus supporting long-term health and preventing disorders related to intestinal dysbiosis.

These natural remedies offer an integrated and holistic approach to boosting the immune system, helping to maintain optimal balance and prevent disease. Adopting these herbs, nutrients, and functional foods can promote a more efficient and sustainable immune response, which is in line with the principles of balance and harmony promoted by ancient traditions and confirmed by modern scientific research.

The Power of Alkaline Fasting in Autoimmune Diseases

Alkaline fasting refers to a controlled period in which you drastically reduce your intake of solid food, giving your body time to rest and regenerate, while continuing to maintain hydration, preferably with alkaline water. This approach does not mean complete abstention from liquids but rather the temporary elimination of foods that can load the system with toxins and acidifying residues, thus promoting a cleaner and more balanced indoor environment.

During fasting, the body does not receive a constant supply of nutrients, allowing the digestive system to rest and the organs to focus on detoxification and cell regeneration. However, this state of absence of concentrated food is extremely delicate and can lead to side effects, such as headaches, dizziness, a drop in blood pressure, and various swerves. For this reason, it is essential to undertake a controlled fast only under the supervision of an expert to monitor for any signs of discomfort and intervene promptly.

Suppose symptoms such as those described above occur during fasting. In that case, it is advisable to temporarily break the fast by introducing a small number of natural sugars, such as honey or fruit, or to resort to drinks containing mineral salts and sugars, such as a solution prepared with water, sugar, and a pinch of salt. These blends help to quickly restore energy balance and normalize blood pressure levels without compromising the benefits of the fasting phase. For diabetic people, it is essential to adopt similar solutions formulated so as not to cause glycemic peaks, using natural sources of sugars with a low glycemic index and specific drinks rich in electrolytes.

Alkaline fasting, if well managed, can positively affect autoimmune diseases, reducing inflammation and allowing the body to cleanse itself of toxins that can trigger incorrect immune reactions. This approach fits perfectly with Dr. Sebi's philosophy, which advocated the importance of keeping the body in an alkaline state through natural nutrition and proper detoxification. According to Dr. Sebi, eliminating processed and acidifying foods and promoting practices such as intermittent fasting under medical supervision can help restore internal balance, strengthen the immune system, and prevent the development of autoimmune diseases. In this way, alkaline fasting becomes a powerful tool to rid the body of metabolic stress and promote long-lasting health, offering a natural and sustainable solution for those who want to take care of their well-being in an integrated way.

Numerous scientific studies have examined the effectiveness of fasting, especially in an alkaline diet, highlighting how this practice can lead to several benefits for metabolic health and body pH balance. Several academic publications have found that intermittent fasting, supplemented with a diet based on natural and alkalizing foods, can help reduce chronic inflammation, improve insulin sensitivity, and promote cell regeneration.

An article published in *Cell Metabolism* highlighted how intermittent fasting induces profound metabolic changes, including an increase in the production of ketones, which act as an alternative energy source and have an anti-inflammatory effect. This study showed how the absence of food for controlled periods allows the body to activate repair mechanisms, reducing oxidative stress and promoting better mitochondrial function. In addition, the benefits of fasting are not limited to the simple process of reducing calorie intake. Still, they are closely linked to the body's ability to "cleanse" itself of accumulated toxins, thanks to the stimulation of autophagia processes, i.e., the removal of damaged cellular components.

Other studies published in the *Journal of Nutrition* and Scientific *Reports* have delved into the effect of fasting on the body's pH balance. An alkaline diet, characterized by the predominant intake of fruits, vegetables, legumes, and whole grains, helps maintain a less acidic internal environment, reducing the production of acidifying metabolic waste. Fasting, integrated in this context, allows the body to use fat reserves as an energy source and promotes greater effectiveness in removing toxins, thus creating a more favorable environment for cell regeneration. This evidence suggests that fasting, combined with an alkaline diet, can effectively improve overall health and prevent chronic diseases, particularly those related to inflammatory processes and metabolic dysfunctions.

In addition, an article published in *JAMA Internal Medicine* highlighted how intermittent fasting can contribute to better weight management and reduced insulin resistance, two key factors in preventing metabolic diseases such as type II diabetes and hypertension. The study showed that alternating fasting and mindful eating induce periods of the body to modulate insulin production more effectively, reducing the metabolic load and facilitating the recovery of hormonal balances.

Finally, research in behavioral nutrition has highlighted how fasting, if followed with caution and under supervision, can also improve psychological well-being, reducing stress and promoting a sense of greater control over one's health. This is especially important given that chronic stress is known to alter immune function and contribute to inflammatory processes that can aggravate numerous chronic conditions.

Current scientific literature supports the idea that fasting and an alkaline diet can bring significant metabolic, inflammatory, and cellular benefits. These studies show how the absence of food for controlled periods allows the body to activate autophagy and regeneration mechanisms, improving metabolism efficiency, reducing oxidative stress, and stabilizing insulin production. These findings represent an essential step towards a deeper understanding of detoxification and cell regeneration processes, offering a natural and sustainable approach to improving long-term health.

Stress Management Techniques to Reduce Autoimmune Crises

Chronic stress, understood as prolonged exposure to emotional, physical, and environmental stressors, is recognized as one of the primary triggers of autoimmune diseases. When the body is subjected to stress for prolonged periods, the production of cortisol and other stress hormones increases steadily. This state of continuous activation leads to a dysfunction of the immune system, as stress hormones, in excess, alter the normal balance between immune cells. As a result, the system cannot correctly distinguish between harmless substances and pathogens, causing inappropriately aggressive reactions against healthy tissues. This process, which manifests as a persistent inflammatory response, progressively damages tissues and reduces the body's ability to repair and regenerate damaged cells.

In addition to directly contributing to the development of autoimmune reactions, chronic stress acts as an amplifier of systemic inflammation, creating an internal environment that further favors the progression of chronic diseases. In this context, autoimmune symptoms intensify, and the body becomes increasingly vulnerable to internal attacks, compromising overall health and quality of life.

This is where Dr. Sebi's revolutionary proposal comes in, who argued that restoring internal balance through an alkaline diet and using natural remedies can be the miracle solution to counteract the deleterious effects of chronic stress. According to Dr. Sebi, eliminating acidifying and toxin-rich foods and replacing them with natural and alkalizing foods allows the body to substantially cleanse itself and reduce inflammation. This holistic approach, which also integrates stress management techniques and medicinal herbs, helps to rebalance the immune system, allowing the body to operate more efficiently and protect it from autoimmune attacks. Dr. Sebi's philosophy is not limited to treating symptoms. Still, it aims to address the root causes of discomfort, offering a long-lasting and natural solution to fight autoimmune diseases. By adopting a nature-focused dietary approach and lifestyle, oxidative stress can be significantly reduced, and cell regeneration can be promoted, thus creating the ideal conditions for a strong and balanced immune system.

Techniques to reduce stress

- **Meditation:** Take a few minutes daily to practice mindfulness or guided meditation. These techniques help calm the mind, reduce cortisol levels, and improve mindfulness by promoting deep relaxation.
- **Deep Breathing:** Breathing exercises, such as diaphragmatic breathing, help slow down the heartbeat and stimulate the parasympathetic system, which promotes relaxation and reduces accumulated tension.
- **Yoga:** The practice of yoga combines physical movements, stretching, and meditation. It improves flexibility, reduces stress, and promotes balance between mind and body. It is particularly effective in reducing anxiety and promoting calmness.
- **Tai Chi:** This ancient Chinese martial art, characterized by slow and fluid movements, helps to improve balance and concentration and reduce stress. It also promotes optimal circulation and deep relaxation.
- **Stretching Exercises:** Regular stretching exercises help release accumulated muscle tension, improve circulation, and facilitate relaxation, thus reducing the symptoms of chronic stress.
- **Regular Physical Activity:** Even simple activities such as walking, light running, or cycling can help reduce stress, stimulate the release of endorphins, and improve cardiovascular health, supporting better physical stress management.
- Relaxation Techniques: Methods such as autogenic training, biofeedback, or guided visualization can teach you how to control your body's response to stress, helping to decrease tension levels and improve mental and physical well-being.
- **Hobbies and Leisure Activities:** Engaging in personal passions and creative pursuits – such as reading, music, gardening, or other forms of art – allows you to take your mind off sources of stress and foster a deep sense of satisfaction and relaxation.
- **Social Support:** Interacting with friends, family, or support groups provides an important emotional outlet. Sharing experiences and feelings can reduce feelings of isolation and provide the necessary support to cope with periods of prolonged stress.

Strategies to eliminate toxins from the body

The human body is constantly exposed to toxins from external sources and internal metabolic processes. External toxins include chemicals in agricultural pesticides, environmental pollutants such as fine particles and exhaust gases, heavy metals that can seep into water and soil, industrial products, and food additives in many processed foods. These substances, accumulated over time, can have deleterious effects on cells, tissues, and organs, compromising the normal functioning of the body and increasing the risk of chronic diseases.

At the same time, our body produces internal toxins due to a dysfunctional metabolism. These include the accumulation of acid waste, the formation of free radicals, and excessive mucus production. These substances are often the result of an unbalanced diet, a sedentary lifestyle, and chronic stress, which push the body to react with constant inflammatory processes. Dr. Sebi argued that this buildup of internal toxins was one of the main culprits of many chronic ailments, as it creates an acidified internal environment that promotes systemic inflammation and reduces the immune system's ability to defend the body.

Thanks to advances in science and medicine, we now better understand the role that the accumulation of toxins plays in compromising health: it can cause widespread inflammation, alterations in metabolism, and reduced immune system efficiency. This continuous accumulation, if not adequately eliminated, becomes unsustainable physiologically and economically as medical expenses and pharmacological treatments to counteract the consequences of these toxins grow exponentially.

Precisely for this reason, more and more research and studies are leading to the rediscovery and integration of natural remedies to fight and eliminate toxins from our bodies. These natural approaches focus on purifying the body through dietary strategies, detox techniques, and medicinal herbs that stimulate waste-elimination processes, reduce inflammation, and promote cell regeneration. This philosophy aims not only to treat symptoms but to intervene in the root causes of toxic accumulation, promoting lasting well-being and reducing dependence on expensive and potentially harmful drug treatments.

Purifying and alkaline power supply

A diet based on whole foods, fruits, vegetables, and legumes is one of the pillars for those who want to take care of family health naturally and effectively. Minimizing processed foods, high in refined sugars and saturated fats, helps keep the body's pH more balanced, promoting the natural elimination of toxins and improving digestion. This dietary approach, strongly supported by Dr. Sebi's philosophy, reduces inflammation levels and creates an internal environment conducive to cell regeneration. For the buyer looking for healthy and simple solutions, including more fruit and vegetables in daily meals is a concrete step to improve energy and prevent disorders related to excess acidity.

Intermittent fasting and controlled detox

Intermittent fasting, if adopted with balance, can be a valuable ally for women and mothers who want a natural method to purify themselves without sacrificing a dynamic lifestyle. This practice involves controlled periods in which the body abstains from solid food, allowing the digestive and metabolic systems to "rest" and activate autophagia processes, i.e., removing damaged cells and toxins. For those who manage a family, it may be helpful to follow intermittent fasting under the supervision of a professional to monitor any side effects and, if necessary, introduce small supplements of natural nutrients (such as purifying herbal teas or vegetable broths) to support the body during periods of food abstinence.

Constant hydration

Maintaining adequate hydration is essential to promote the body's detoxification since water facilitates the elimination of waste through urine and sweat. Those who take care of the whole family's needs can make hydration more pleasant and healthy by adding lemon or ginger to the water to enhance the anti-inflammatory and purifying effect. This habit is easy to adopt keep a bottle or carafe handy, perhaps in the kitchen or on the worktable, remember to drink regularly, and maintain a cleaner indoor environment less prone to toxins accumulation.

Purifying infusions and herbal teas

Integrating herbal teas such as dandelion, milk thistle, or other purifying plants into your daily routine is an easy and natural method to support the liver, kidneys, and the entire digestive system in removing waste. When consumed consistently, these infusions stimulate diuresis and reduce the toxic load, improving metabolic function and contributing to a less inflamed internal environment. For the buyer looking for solutions suitable for the whole family, herbal teas can become a moment of shared relaxation, ideal for offering during afternoon breaks or after dinner.

Regular exercise and sweat-inducing activities

Regular physical activities like walking, light running, yoga, or even simple sauna sessions help maintain an active metabolism and reduce stress levels. Constant movement, in fact, stimulates blood and lymphatic circulation, promoting the elimination of toxins through sweat. Those with little time can opt for half-hour walks a day or short yoga sessions early in the morning or before bedtime. This way, exercise becomes a natural part of the family routine, improving tissue oxygenation and overall psychophysical well-being.

Support with antioxidant herbs

Herbs rich in antioxidant compounds, such as turmeric, ginger, and green tea, play a key role in neutralizing free radicals produced by metabolism. This is especially important for women who want to take care of their skin, prevent signs of aging, and strengthen the family's immune system. Regular intake of these herbs, in the form of herbal teas or added to meals, can reduce inflammation and promote better cell regeneration, making the body more resistant to environmental stressors.

Reduction of exposure to environmental toxins

In addition to changing your diet and lifestyle, limiting contact with toxic environmental substances, such as pesticides, air pollutants, heavy metals, and household chemicals, is essential. Choosing household cleaning and personal hygiene products with natural ingredients, preferring organic foods, and washing fruit and vegetables thoroughly are small precautions that, added together, contribute to maintaining a cleaner indoor environment. By doing so, the workload of the body's elimination system is lightened, promoting long-lasting health and excellent protection for the whole family.

Autoimmune diseases are conditions in which the immune system mistakenly attacks healthy tissues instead of protecting the body. Understanding their nature is essential, as these diseases often have deep roots in chronic inflammation, the imbalance of the intestinal barrier, and the accumulation of toxins, factors that, interacting with each other, compromise the well-being of the body. Knowing these mechanisms allows us to address autoimmune diseases in a targeted way, intervening on the underlying causes of the problem and not just treating the symptoms.

To effectively and naturally combat these conditions, adopting a holistic approach that integrates an alkaline diet, medicinal herbs and natural remedies, detox techniques, and stress management strategies is essential. A proper diet rich in whole foods, fruits, vegetables, and legumes promotes a less acidified internal environment, reducing inflammation and strengthening the immune system. Natural remedies, such as the specific herbs we've looked at, help to modulate the immune response and protect the body from autoimmune reactions. At the same time, controlled fasting and stress management techniques offer the body a chance to repair, regenerate, and restore a balance critical for long-lasting health.

Dr. Sebi's philosophy emphasizes the importance of living in harmony with nature, adopting a lifestyle that is not only based on natural and purifying nutrition but also embraces detox practices, physical exercise, and relaxation techniques. According to Dr. Sebi, giving back to the body what nature offers in pure, unprocessed form allows toxins to be eliminated, inflammation reduced, and immune defenses strengthened, leading to a state of well-being reflected in increased energy, vitality, and zest for life.

Understanding the nature of autoimmune diseases and adopting natural and holistic strategies to combat them is an essential step towards a healthier and more energized life. Embracing Dr. Sebi's approach means investing in one's health in a sustainable and lasting way, recognizing that well-being is not just the absence of disease but a state of physical, mental, and emotional balance that allows us to live each day with vitality and joy.

CHAPTER 12. DR SEBI AND THYROID DISORDERS

The thyroid is a critically crucial endocrine gland that regulates the metabolism and energy of the entire body through the production of hormones such as thyroxine (T4) and triiodothyronine (T3). Thyroid disorders, which manifest as hypothyroidism or hyperthyroidism, can have a profound impact not only on metabolism but also on mood, energy level, and overall quality of life. In recent years, the growing attention to natural and holistic approaches has led to a rediscovery of the role of nutrition and natural remedies, as proposed by Dr. Sebi, in supporting and rebalancing thyroid function.

A key point of this approach is the alkaline diet, which is based on the intake of natural, whole, and plant-based foods. This diet can maintain a balanced pH within the body. According to Dr. Sebi, a less acidified environment promotes cell regeneration and reduces inflammation, two essential elements for proper thyroid functioning. A cleansing and alkaline diet can help improve cellular sensitivity to thyroid hormones and provide vital nutrients in metabolism.

The correct balance of essential minerals, such as iodine, selenium, zinc, and iron, is crucial for a healthy thyroid. These micronutrients support the synthesis of thyroid hormones but also help protect the gland's cells from oxidative and inflammatory damage. Dr. Sebi's proposed diet encourages the consumption of foods rich in these minerals, such as green leafy vegetables, fruits, nuts, and seeds, while suggesting avoiding processed foods and chemical additives that can compromise mineral balance.

Another important aspect is the role of alkaline herbs, especially Fucus Vesiculosus, a seaweed rich in iodine and other minerals, which, according to Dr. Sebi, help stimulate thyroid function naturally. Thanks to their anti-inflammatory and antioxidant properties, other herbs help create an internal environment conducive to thyroid health, reducing oxidative stress and improving the circulation of essential nutrients.

Managing thyroid disorders is not only limited to proper nutrient intake but also involves a thorough understanding of foods to avoid. For example, for those suffering from hypothyroidism or hyperthyroidism, it is essential to limit the consumption of foods and substances that can interfere with thyroid function, such as highly processed foods, excess soy, and certain types of shellfish, which can contain high levels of goitrogenic substances.

Another crucial element is the link between stress, adrenaline, and thyroid health. Chronic stress induces the release of adrenaline and cortisol, hormones that, in excess, can impair the normal functioning of the thyroid, altering metabolism and worsening symptoms of thyroid dysfunction. Stress management techniques, such as meditation, yoga, and deep breathing, become valuable tools for maintaining hormonal balance and supporting thyroid function.

Natural remedies to improve metabolism and energy play a fundamental integrative role. A well-functioning metabolism is the foundation for an energy-filled life, and natural approaches, which include cleansing foods, stimulating herbs, and detox practices, can help optimize thyroid function and improve quality of life. Dr. Sebi's approach, emphasizing natural, cleansing, and alkaline nutrition, offers a complete solution for those who want to tackle thyroid disorders sustainably and naturally, promoting well-being, energy, and a greater desire to live.

This chapter will explore in detail how the alkaline diet, essential minerals, specific herbs such as Fucus Vesiculosus, conscious choice of foods to avoid, stress management, and natural remedies can work together to rebalance thyroid function, improve metabolism, and support the body's overall vitality.

How the alkaline diet can rebalance thyroid function

The alkaline diet is based on the predominant intake of natural, whole, and plant-based foods to keep the body's pH slightly alkaline. This approach is particularly beneficial for the health of the thyroid, a critical gland that regulates metabolism, energy, and the functioning of numerous organs. When the body operates in a less acidified environment, inflammation, and oxidative stress are reduced, conditions that could otherwise impair thyroid function and damage cells. A crucial aspect of this dietary approach is the optimal intake of essential minerals such as iodine, selenium, and zinc, which play critical roles in producing and regulating thyroid hormones.

Iodine is an essential component for the synthesis of thyroid hormones T3 and T4. Without adequate amounts of iodine, the thyroid gland cannot produce enough hormones, leading to hypothyroidism. Natural sources of iodine include seaweed, Brazil nuts, and fish. Although plant foods are usually preferred in the alkaline diet, it is essential to supplement this mineral through natural sources or supplements, always under medical supervision.

Selenium is key in converting inactive thyroid hormone (T4) into active thyroid hormone (T3). It is also known for its antioxidant properties, which protect the thyroid gland from oxidative damage. The presence of selenoproteins is essential for proper thyroid functioning, and its deficiency can lead to reduced metabolic efficiency and an increased risk of autoimmune diseases. The primary plant sources of selenium include Brazil nuts, sunflower seeds, and whole grains, all of which are ideally suited to the alkaline diet approach.

Zinc is another essential mineral for thyroid health. It intervenes in synthesizing hormones and the immune system's functioning. Zinc helps maintain the structure and enzyme activity necessary for thyroid hormone metabolism and protects against oxidative stress. A diet rich in whole foods, such as legumes, nuts, and seeds, provides zinc in adequate quantities and contributes to optimal assimilation of this mineral, thus naturally supporting thyroid function.

Adopting an alkaline diet, therefore, means limiting the intake of processed foods and acidifiers and favoring foods that provide these essential minerals. This approach helps to ensure that the thyroid can produce hormones in optimal quantity and quality, contributing to the proper functioning of metabolism and cell regeneration. Essentially, a well-balanced alkaline diet promotes a less inflamed and more nutrient-rich internal environment, which is the foundation of an efficient thyroid system and long-lasting overall well-being.

Antioxidants and thyroid health

Antioxidant compounds play a crucial role in protecting the thyroid from oxidative stress. This process can impair gland function and trigger cell damage. Antioxidants neutralize free radicals, unstable molecules produced during metabolism that, if left unchecked, can damage thyroid cells and interfere with the production of hormones essential for the proper functioning of metabolism. Antioxidant-rich foods, such as leafy greens and fruits, berries, citrus fruits, and nuts, offer natural protection against oxidative stress. In addition, natural supplements such as green tea and turmeric, thanks to the presence of compounds such as catechins and curcumin, promote thyroid cell regeneration and help maintain hormonal balance. Numerous studies, such as those published in *The Journal of Clinical Endocrinology & Metabolism*, show that an adequate intake of antioxidants is related to better thyroid function and a reduction in oxidative damage, demonstrating the importance of these compounds for endocrine health.

Holistic approach in the management of thyroid disorders

A holistic approach to managing thyroid disorders considers the body as an integrated system in which nutrition, physical activity, stress management, and natural remedies work synergistically to restore internal balance. In this context, it is not enough to treat the symptoms. Still, intervening in the root causes, such as inflammation, oxidative stress, and nutritional imbalances, is essential. Supplementing a cleansing, alkaline diet rich in whole foods and important minerals, detox techniques, and using medicinal herbs, such as Fucus Vesiculosus, can significantly improve thyroid function. In parallel, regular physical activity and relaxation techniques, such as meditation and yoga, help reduce chronic stress, a known trigger for endocrine dysfunction. This holistic approach, supported by numerous scientific studies and in line with Dr. Sebi's philosophy, promotes a more efficient thyroid and overall well-being that translates into increased energy, emotional stability, and quality of life. Adopting this integrated vision makes it possible to address thyroid disorders naturally and sustainably, promoting cell regeneration and hormonal balance with a view to long-term health.

Physical activity and thyroid

Regular physical activity is key to boosting metabolism and supporting the functioning of the endocrine system, including the thyroid. When we practice moderate physical exercise, such as walking, light running, yoga, and stretching sessions, we promote better blood and lymphatic circulation. This helps thyroid hormones reach all cells in the body more efficiently, optimizing metabolism and energy utilization.

Yoga, for example, improves flexibility, reduces muscle tension, and affects the nervous system. By reducing levels of cortisol, the stress hormone, yoga promotes emotional balance that has a positive effect on metabolism and, consequently, thyroid function. Similarly, resistance exercises, such as light weightlifting or bodyweight exercises (e.g., squats and push-ups), stimulate muscle growth. Increased muscle mass increases the body's ability to use glucose as an energy source, essential for maintaining proper hormonal balance.

Several studies published in the *Diabetes & Metabolism Journal* have shown that those who exercise regularly show better control of blood sugar levels and increased insulin sensitivity, which are indirect benefits that support thyroid function.

Here are some recommended activities include:

- **Regular walks:** Ideal for those with a busy lifestyle and looking for a low-impact activity.
- **Yoga and stretching:** Perfect for improving flexibility and reducing stress, contributing to a mind-body balance.
- **Light running or jogging** is a good option to stimulate metabolism and increase cardiovascular endurance.
- **Cycling:** Suitable for both indoor and outdoor exercisers, cycling helps improve circulation and reduce stress.
- **Swimming** is a low-impact physical activity that promotes optimal circulation and strengthens the cardiovascular system.

Incorporating these sports into your daily routine can promote better thyroid function, contributing to a more efficient metabolism, optimal glycemic control, and overall well-being in line with an active and healthy lifestyle.

Essential minerals for a healthy thyroid

Thyroid health is closely linked to the balanced supply of essential minerals, which play a key role in producing and regulating thyroid hormones. These nutrients support hormone synthesis, protect thyroid cells from oxidative stress, and help maintain an efficient metabolism. Below is a list of the main minerals to consider for a healthy thyroid, with a brief description of their benefits and food sources:

- **Iodine:** Iodine is essential for producing thyroid hormones T3 and T4. An iodine deficiency can lead to hypothyroidism and the formation of goiters. Food sources rich in iodine include seaweed, fish, dairy products, and sometimes, iodized salt.
- **Selenium:** Selenium's antioxidant properties make it essential for converting the inactive hormone T4 into the active hormone T3 and protecting the thyroid from oxidative damage. It is found in Brazil nuts, sunflower seeds, whole grains, and fish.
- **Zinc:** Zinc plays a key role in synthesizing thyroid hormones and modulating the immune system. Proper zinc intake also supports enzyme function and cellular metabolism. Good sources of zinc include legumes, nuts, seeds, whole grains, and some leafy greens.
- **Iron:** Iron is vital for energy production, oxygen transport, and the proper functioning of metabolism. An iron deficiency can indirectly affect thyroid function and overall health. The primary sources of iron include legumes, spinach, seeds, nuts, and whole grains.
- **Magnesium** is crucial for numerous biochemical processes, including regulating energy metabolism and maintaining muscle and nerve function. It helps maintain hormonal balance and protect the thyroid from oxidative stress. It is abundant in nuts, seeds, leafy greens, legumes, and whole grains.

Maintaining an adequate balance of these minerals through a varied and balanced diet is essential for adequately functioning the thyroid gland and preventing dysfunctions that can negatively affect metabolism and general well-being. If necessary, targeted supplements should always be evaluated by a health professional to ensure that the body is receiving the right amount of these essential nutrients.

The role of Fucus Vesiculosus and other alkaline herbs

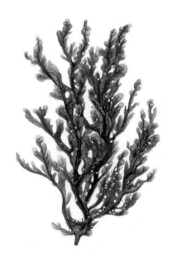

Fucus vesiculosus, commonly known as sponge seaweed or bladderwrack, is a brown seaweed that grows in the cold waters of the Atlantic and Northern Europe. Used for centuries in traditional medicines, Fucus is particularly prized for its high content of iodine and other essential minerals, making it a valuable ally in supporting thyroid function. In the context of an alkaline diet, Fucus vesiculosus and other alkaline herbs are considered effective tools for restoring internal balance, reducing inflammation and promoting cell regeneration, which are crucial for thyroid health.

Fucus vesiculosus is rich in various phytoactive ingredients that determine its beneficial properties. Among these, **iodine content** is crucial: iodine is essential for the synthesis of thyroid hormones T3 and T4, and Fucus provides a natural and bioavailable source of this mineral, helping to maintain optimal thyroid function. In addition, Fucus contains **fucoidans**, polysaccharides found in the cell walls of brown algae, which have demonstrated anti-inflammatory and immunomodulatory properties. Fucoidans can help reduce oxidative stress at the cellular level, protecting the thyroid from damage and improving tissue regeneration.

Another important group of compounds found in Fucus are **polyphenols**, which are known for their powerful antioxidant effect. These compounds help neutralize free radicals, helping to maintain pH balance and reduce chronic inflammation, two factors that can impair thyroid function. The **alginates** present in the seaweed also promote the elimination of toxins and improve nutrient absorption, supporting metabolism and the overall health of the endocrine system.

In addition to Fucus, other alkaline herbs play a complementary role in supporting thyroid function. For example, herbs such as **dandelion** and **milk thistle** not only promote the purification of the liver and kidneys, but help to create a less acidified internal environment, promoting the absorption of essential minerals and reducing inflammation. These herbs, together with Fucus, are an effective combination to restore harmony to the endocrine system and support the optimal production of thyroid hormones.

Fucus vesiculosus, thanks to its phytoactive ingredients such as iodine, fucoidans, polyphenols and alginates, is a powerful natural remedy for thyroid health. Its ability to provide essential minerals, protect cells from oxidative damage and promote the purification of the body makes it particularly suitable in an alkaline diet regimen. Integrated with other purifying and adaptogenic herbs, Fucus helps to create an internal environment conducive to cell regeneration, the reduction of inflammation and the maintenance of optimal thyroid function, in line with Dr. Sebi's philosophy for long-lasting and natural well-being.

Foods to Avoid with Hypothyroidism and Hyperthyroidism

Foods to avoid for those suffering from hypothyroidism and hyperthyroidism are crucial in preventing the worsening of thyroid disorders and maintaining a stable hormonal balance. Inadequate consumption of certain foods can, in fact, aggravate thyroid function, altering the production of T3 and T4 and increasing inflammation, with possible consequences such as weight gain, fatigue, irritability, and cardiovascular problems.

High-sodium foods and excess table salt are the first hurdle to preserving thyroid health. Sodium abuse, in fact, promotes water retention and increases blood volume, increasing blood pressure and subjecting the cardiovascular system to more significant stress. This overload can negatively affect hormone production, especially in individuals prone to thyroid imbalances. Reducing salt consumption and preferring aromatic herbs and natural spices to flavor dishes become recommended choices for those who want to protect their thyroid and heart health. Processed and convenience foods are second-critical elements, as they often contain high sodium levels, additives, and preservatives that can contribute to a chronic inflammatory state. This inflammation, in turn, can impair the production of thyroid hormones and promote autoimmune reactions, which is particularly dangerous for those already struggling with thyroid-related disorders. For the buyer person attentive to family health, it is essential to replace ready meals with home-cooked meals, preferably based on fresh and whole foods, to reduce the introduction of potentially harmful chemicals and preservatives. Soy products are another group of foods to watch, as they contain goitrogenic compounds that can interfere with the absorption of iodine, a mineral essential for synthesizing thyroid hormones. This is particularly relevant for hypothyroidism, where the gland produces fewer hormones, and hyperthyroidism, where the gland is overactive. To avoid further hormonal imbalance, the buyer who wants vegetarian or vegan options must pay attention to the quantities of soy consumed, favoring alternative protein sources such as legumes, whole grains, and oilseeds.

Foods high in refined sugars and carbohydrates with a high glycemic index are an additional danger, as they can cause glycemic spikes and increase insulin production. In the long run, this condition impairs hormonal balance and promotes an inflammatory state, worsening thyroid disorders. For those who run a family and want to offer healthy food choices, replacing industrial sweets with fresh fruit and opting for whole grains instead of refined flour is essential. This will keep blood sugar levels stable and protect the thyroid. High-fat dairy products, such as aged cheeses or whole milk, can increase systemic inflammation and interfere with hormonal balance, making it more challenging to maintain optimal thyroid function. Buyer personas looking for lighter alternatives, such as skimmed milk, plant-based drinks, or low-fat yogurts, can thus contain inflammation and offer the family a more balanced diet, especially for those predisposed to thyroid problems. Fried foods and industrial snacks are an additional category to avoid, as they are rich in trans and saturated fats that increase inflammation and alter lipid metabolism. This process makes it more complicated to control hormone levels, especially in those suffering from hypothyroidism or hyperthyroidism. Choosing healthier cooking methods, such as steaming, baking, or grilling, helps preserve the quality of your food and limit your intake of harmful fats. Sugary drinks and sodas pose an additional risk, as they contain added sugars that increase calorie intake in an unwanted way, promoting glycemic spikes and inflammation. In the long run, this condition can negatively affect thyroid function and hinder energy and hormonal recovery. Preferring water, herbal teas, or vegetable drinks without added sugar helps maintain a stable metabolic profile and reduces the overall toxic load.

Avoiding these foods is crucial as excessive intake of acidifying and processed foods compromise the body's pH balance, increases systemic inflammation, and hinders the absorption of essential nutrients, such as iodine, necessary for producing thyroid hormones. In addition, a diet rich in processed products and poor-quality fats accentuates oxidative stress. It promotes the accumulation of toxins, further damaging the thyroid and aggravating symptoms in both hypothyroidism and hyperthyroidism. Adopting a diet free of these foods and replacing them with more natural, whole, and alkaline alternatives can significantly help improve thyroid function, reduce inflammation, and promote more balanced and long-lasting overall well-being.

The Link between Stress, adrenaline, and thyroid health

Chronic stress and the constant production of adrenaline are two factors that significantly affect thyroid health. When the body is subjected to prolonged stress, response mechanisms are activated, leading to high production of hormones such as cortisol and adrenaline. If released in excess, these hormones can disrupt hormonal balance and interfere with normal thyroid function. High adrenaline levels can lead to vasoconstriction, reducing blood circulation and hindering the proper transport of thyroid hormones at the cellular level. This state of constant alert not only speeds up metabolism but can also trigger a chronic inflammatory cycle that damages thyroid cells in the long run, impairing their ability to produce essential hormones such as T3 and T4. As a result, chronic stress and the associated production of adrenaline not only worsen thyroid function but also promote the onset of metabolic and autoimmune disorders, negatively affecting general well-being.

Dr. Sebi's philosophy is based on a holistic approach to health, recognizing the interconnectedness of mind, body, and environment. According to Dr. Sebi, one of the fundamental steps to keep the thyroid optimal is to reduce stress and control adrenaline levels through a natural, purifying, and alkaline diet. He argued that a balanced internal environment, free from toxins and acidifying foods, allows the body to function more efficiently, reducing the need to produce excess stress hormones. Through a diet rich in whole foods, fruits, vegetables, and legumes, you foster an alkaline environment that supports thyroid function and helps mitigate chronic stress's effects. In addition, Dr. Sebi encouraged using herbs and natural remedies, such as holy basil (Tulsi) and other adaptogenic herbs, to calm the nervous system and lower adrenaline levels. This integrated approach combines a natural diet with stress management practices, reduces the inflammatory load, promotes cell regeneration, and keeps the thyroid in optimal health, thus promoting overall well-being and increased energy to face daily challenges.

Natural remedies to improve metabolism and energy

1. **Fucus Vesiculosus** — This herb can be taken in herbal tea: a teaspoon of Fucus vesiculosus dried in 250 ml of boiling water for 10 minutes, then filtered. Rich in iodine and essential minerals, it supports the production of thyroid hormones, stimulates metabolism, cleanses the body, and promotes an alkaline internal environment, helping to improve energy.

2. **Dandelion** – An herbal tea made from a teaspoon of dried root in 250 ml of boiling water for 10 minutes helps detoxify the liver and kidneys, reducing the accumulation of toxins. It improves digestion and metabolism, increasing energy and more efficient thyroid function.
3. **Milk thistle** – A teaspoon of crushed seeds in 250 ml of boiling water, left to simmer for 10 minutes, then filtered, provides silymarin, which protects and regenerates liver cells. A cleansed liver indirectly supports the thyroid and metabolism, improving energy efficiency and resistance to oxidative stress.
4. **Ashwagandha (Withania somnifera)** can be consumed in tea (one teaspoon of dried root in 250 ml of boiling water for 5-7 minutes) or in powdered form. This adaptogenic herb regulates cortisol levels, reduces stress, and improves hormonal balance. It promotes a more efficient metabolism and increased energy and directly supports thyroid health.
5. **Turmeric** – Half a teaspoon of turmeric powder in 250 ml of boiling water or unsweetened plant milk, left to infuse for 5-10 minutes, protects thyroid cells from oxidative stress. Thanks to curcumin, this translates into a more active metabolism and a higher energy level.
6. **Ginseng (Panax ginseng)** – A decoction with a teaspoon of dried root in 250 ml of boiling water, simmered for 10 minutes, improves energy and physical endurance due to its stimulating and adaptogenic effect. It promotes an active metabolism and increased insulin sensitivity, contributing to the well-being of the thyroid.
7. **Tulsi (Holy Basil)** - An herbal tea made by soaking a teaspoon of dried leaves in 250 ml of boiling water for 5-7 minutes helps reduce stress and promote hormonal balance. A less stressed immune system and better stress management support thyroid function and boost overall energy.
8. **Ginger** – A tea with 3-4 slices of fresh root in 250 ml of boiling water for 5-7 minutes improves digestion, stimulates circulation, and facilitates the transport of essential nutrients. Its anti-inflammatory and thermogenic properties promote fat-burning and support thyroid function, keeping energy levels high.
9. **Olives and Extra Virgin Olive Oil** – Consume fresh olives as a snack or use them to dress salads. At the same time, the oil is ideal for cooking at low temperatures or as a raw condiment. Rich in antioxidants and healthy fats, they promote controlled inflammation, support immune function, and protect cells from oxidative stress, maintaining a balanced metabolism, which is crucial for thyroid health.
10. **Aloe Vera** – Pure juice, diluted in water or added to smoothies, promotes cell regeneration and soothes inflammation, improving nutrient absorption and gut health. A healthy gut is crucial for a balanced immune system and proper thyroid hormone metabolism.
11. **Probiotics and Prebiotics** – Supplementing fermented foods such as natural yogurt, kefir, sauerkraut, and kimchi, along with sources of prebiotics (garlic, onion, bananas, asparagus, chicory root), maintains a healthy gut microbiota, which is essential for regulating the immune system and metabolism. A balanced gut improves nutrient absorption and supports thyroid function, contributing to overall well-being.
12. **Vitamin C (from natural sources)** – Fresh citrus fruits such as oranges, lemons, kiwis, strawberries, or freshly prepared juices and smoothies provide a powerful antioxidant that protects cells from oxidative stress and promotes tissue regeneration. An adequate intake of vitamin C strengthens the immune system. It supports the synthesis of thyroid hormones, promoting a healthy metabolism and long-lasting energy. These natural remedies, included in a balanced diet and an active lifestyle, offer valuable support to improve thyroid function, stimulate metabolism, and increase energy levels. Adopting these strategies allows you to achieve a better hormonal balance, protect cells from oxidative stress, and promote lasting well-being, which aligns with the holistic approach supported by ancient traditions and the latest scientific evidence.

CHAPTER 13: HOW TO BOOST THE IMMUNE SYSTEM

The immune system is our natural shield, a complex set of cells, organs, and processes that protect us from viruses, bacteria, and other external threats. However, prolonged stress conditions, an unbalanced diet, exposure to environmental pollutants, and sedentary lifestyles can weaken these defenses, making us more susceptible to infections and diseases. This chapter will explore how to support and boost the immune system through natural remedies, integrating Dr. Sebi's principles with other traditional and modern knowledge and improving our long-term health.

The first step to a strong immune system is to adopt a diet rich in essential nutrients, such as minerals, vitamins, and antioxidants, that promote cell regeneration and proper communication between immune cells. This is where alkalizing foods and medicinal herbs come into play, from which we can draw active ingredients capable of modulating the immune response and reducing inflammatory processes. This approach is not limited to counteracting the symptoms of any disease. Still, it intervenes at the roots, promoting a balanced internal environment where the body can best express its defense capabilities.

In parallel, considering other aspects of our daily lives, such as sleep, physical activity, and stress management, is crucial, as efficiently affects the immune system's ability to respond to threats. Adequate sleep, for example, is essential for producing cytokines, molecules that regulate inflammation and the immune response. Moderate exercise, on the other hand, improves circulation and helps maintain a healthy body weight, thus preventing complications related to obesity or a sedentary lifestyle. Finally, stress management plays a crucial role: excess cortisol can weaken immune reactivity, paving the way for recurrent infections and chronic inflammation.

In this chapter, we will see how natural remedies and wellness practices can act on several levels to support the body's defenses, from the choice of specific foods and supplements (such as echinacea, astragalus, medicinal mushrooms, and probiotics) to the preparation of herbal teas and juices rich in minerals and vitamins. We will also delve into prevention strategies, including personal hygiene and home care. We will highlight the importance of a holistic approach, considering the relationships between body, mind, and environment.

The goal is to protect oneself from viruses and bacteria and build a solid foundation for general well-being, promoting vitality and longevity. In an era in which exposure to toxic substances and sources of stress is high, rediscovering the power of natural remedies and good habits becomes an act of responsibility towards oneself and one's future health. Through practical advice and suggestions, this chapter offers a complete guide to anyone who wants to adopt a lifestyle in harmony with the principles of nature, maximizing their resistance to disease and living every day with more energy and serenity.

Best Immune-Boosting Herbs

Focusing on plants known for their adaptogenic and anti-inflammatory properties is essential when choosing herbs that can strengthen the immune system.

Echinacea

Echinacea is a plant widely studied for its immune-stimulating properties, particularly its ability to promote the production of white blood cells (lymphocytes and macrophages) involved in the body's defense against viruses and bacteria. In addition to this stimulating effect, echinacea possesses anti-inflammatory properties that help contain inflammatory processes, reducing cold and flu symptoms. It can be taken in herbal tea, mother tincture, or capsules. It is beneficial in the winter or during seasonal changes when the immune system can weaken.

Astragalus

Astragalus is a plant native to traditional Chinese medicine known for its high content of immunomodulating polysaccharides. These compounds help the body regulate the immune response in a balanced way, making them particularly effective during stress and fatigue. Astragalus also helps to strengthen resistance to infection, improving vitality and supporting the body in physical or mental overwork. It is often found as a dried root used in herbal teas, decoctions, capsules, and tablets.

Ashwagandha (Withania somnifera)

Considered a leading adaptogenic herb, ashwagandha helps the body better manage stress by modulating levels of the stress hormone cortisol. By reducing the adverse effects of chronic stress, ashwagandha allows the immune system to function more efficiently. This plant has been used for centuries in Ayurvedic medicine to improve physical endurance, mental energy, and general well-being, promoting a psycho-physical balance that positively impacts the body's ability to defend itself.

Elderberry (flowers and berries)

Elderberry is known for its remarkable antiviral and antioxidant properties. The flowers and berries of this plant contain compounds that can support the body in the fight against seasonal infections, such as colds and flu. The high antioxidant content helps reduce oxidative stress, protecting cells from free radical damage. Elderberry can be taken as herbal tea, syrup, or supplement. It is particularly effective when used at the first signs of discomfort to promote a faster immune response.

Reishi (Ganoderma lucidum)

Reishi is a medicinal mushroom appreciated in many traditions, from Chinese to Japanese medicine, for its ability to modulate the immune response. It acts by reducing inflammatory processes and regulating the activity of immune cells, making it sound both in cases of hyperactivation of the immune system and in conditions of weakness or increased exposure to infections. Rich in polysaccharides and triterpenes, reishi also helps to improve stress resistance and overall vitality.

Infusions and decoctions to strengthen natural defenses.

In addition to taking herbs as capsules or tinctures, preparing infusions and decoctions is a simple and pleasant way to enjoy their properties. Some effective combinations include:

Echinacea + Elderberry

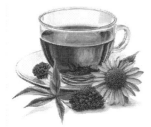

Ingredients

- 1 teaspoon dried echinacea
- 1 teaspoon dried elderflower
- 250 ml boiling water

Guidelines:

1. Bring the water to a boil.
2. Place echinacea and elderflower in a cup.
3. Pour boiling water over the ingredients.
4. Cover and leave to infuse for 5-10 minutes. Filter and drink hot.

Astragalus + Ginger Root

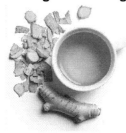

Ingredients

- 1 teaspoon dried astragalus
- 3-4 slices of fresh ginger root
- 300 ml of water

Guidelines:

1. Put the water in a saucepan and add astragalus and ginger.
2. Bring to a boil.
3. Reduce the heat and simmer for 10-15 minutes.
4. Filters and consumes hot.

Ashwagandha + Licorice

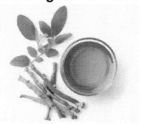

Ingredients

- 1 tsp dried ashwagandha root
- 1 piece of licorice root
- 250 ml boiling water

Guidelines:

1. Heat the water until boiling.
2. Place ashwagandha and licorice in a cup.
3. Pour boiling water over the ingredients.
4. Cover and leave to infuse for 5-10 minutes.
5. Filter and drink in moderation.

Reishi + Rosehip

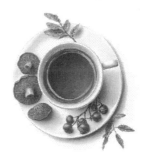

Ingredients:

- 1 teaspoon of reishi powder (or a piece of dried mushroom)
- 1 teaspoon rosehip berries
- 300 ml of water

Guidelines:

1. Pour the water into a saucepan and add the reishi and rose hips.
2. Bring to a boil. Simmer for 10 minutes.
3. Filters and consumes hot.

Tulsi (Holy Basil) + Mint

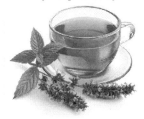

Prep Time: 5 min,
Ingredients:

- 1 teaspoon dried tulsi
- 1 teaspoon dried or fresh mint leaves
- 250 ml boiling water

Guidelines:

1. Bring the water to a boil.
2. Put tulsi and mint in a cup.
3. Pour boiling water over the ingredients.
4. Cover and leave to infuse for 5-8 minutes.
5. Strain and serve hot.

Burdock + Turmeric

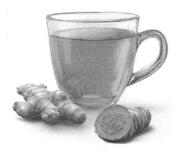

Prep Time: 5 min, Cook Time: 10 min,
Ingredients:

- 1 tsp dried burdock root
- 1/2 teaspoon turmeric powder
- 300 ml of water

Guidelines:

1. Put the water in a saucepan and add the burdock and turmeric.
2. Bring to a boil.
3. Reduce the heat and simmer for 10 minutes.
4. Filters and consumes hot.

Ginseng (Panax ginseng) + Cardamom

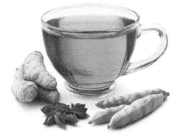

Prep Time: 5 min, Cook Time: 10 min,
Ingredients:

- 1 teaspoon of ginseng powder or 1 piece of dried root
- 2-3 crushed cardamom berries
- 300 ml of water

Guidelines:

1. Pour the water into a saucepan and add the ginseng and cardamom.
2. Bring to a boil.
3. Simmer for 10 minutes.
4. Filter and drink in moderation.

Nettle + Fennel

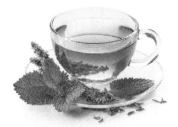

Prep Time: 5 min,
Ingredients:

- 1 teaspoon dried nettle leaves
- 1 teaspoon fennel seeds
- 250 ml boiling water

Guidelines:

1. Bring the water to a boil.
2. Put nettle and fennel seeds in a cup.
3. Pour boiling water over the ingredients.
4. Cover and leave to infuse for 5-8 minutes.
5. Filter and drink.

Sage + Lemon

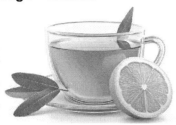

Prep Time: 5 min,
Ingredients:

- 1 teaspoon dried sage leaves
- Juice of 1/2 lemon
- 250 ml boiling water

Guidelines:

1. Bring the water to a boil.
2. Put the sage in a cup and add the lemon juice.
3. Pour in the boiling water.
4. Cover and leave to infuse for 5 minutes.
5. Filters and consumes hot.

Milk thistle + Dandelion

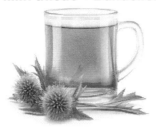

Prep Time: 5 min, Cook Time: 10 min,
Ingredients:

- 1 teaspoon of crushed milk thistle seeds
- 1 teaspoon dried dandelion root
- 300 ml of water

Guidelines:

1. Put the water in a saucepan and add milk thistle and dandelion.
2. Bring to a boil.
3. Reduce the heat and simmer for 10 minutes.
4. Strain and serve hot.

Chamomile + Ginger

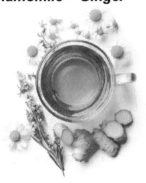

Prep Time: 5 min,
Ingredients

- 1 teaspoon of chamomile flowers
- 3-4 slices of fresh ginger
- 250 ml boiling water

Guidelines

1. Bring the water to a boil.
2. Put the chamomile and ginger in a cup.
3. Pour in the boiling water and cover.
4. Leave to infuse for 5-7 minutes.
5. Filter and drink hot.

Thyme + Manuka Honey

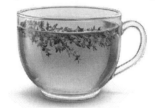

Prep Time: 5 min,
Ingredients:

- 1 teaspoon dried thyme leaves
- 1 teaspoon of Manuka honey (to add to a warm drink)
- 250 ml boiling water

Guidelines:

1. Bring the water to a boil.
2. Place the thyme in a cup.
3. Pour in the boiling water and cover.
4. Leave to infuse for 5 minutes.
5. Filter and wait for the drink to cool down before adding the honey.

Detox routine for the lymphatic system

The lymphatic system is of fundamental importance in eliminating toxins and maintaining efficient immune defenses since, unlike the circulatory system, which can count on the heart's pumping action, the lymph moves thanks to muscle contractions and other external mechanical stimuli. For this reason, adopting a detox routine to improve lymphatic circulation and promote more effective fluid drainage is helpful, especially for those who manage a busy family and work life but still want to devote time to their health. A first recommended practice is dry brushing, which consists of gently massaging the skin with a natural bristle brush, starting from the body's extremities and proceeding towards the heart. This simple gesture, to be performed in the morning or before a shower, stimulates lymphatic flow and promotes waste elimination while giving a feeling of vitality and brighter skin. A second approach involves immersion in a hot bath enriched with Epsom salts, composed mainly of magnesium sulfate, capable of relaxing the muscles and promoting lymphatic circulation thanks to sweating induced by the heat of the water. In addition to reducing accumulated tension and stress, this habit can help rid the body of toxins and waste. Light physical activity is also essential: yoga, tai chi, or simple walks are exercises that, although not particularly intense, promote muscle contraction and, therefore, the push of lymph toward the lymph nodes, where the filtration of waste takes place. Consistently practicing gentle disciplines or walking regularly improves muscle tone and lymphatic circulation, positively affecting water retention and skin appearance. Finally, the intake of draining herbs represents additional support to maintain a cleaner internal environment: birch, dandelion, and nettle, for example, have diuretic and purifying properties that lighten the workload of the lymphatic system, stimulating diuresis and facilitate the elimination of excess fluids. Preparing herbal teas or decoctions with these plants and consuming them regularly, combining adequate hydration, creates a synergistic effect that can further enhance the drainage of toxins. With the adoption of these simple measures, which can be easily included in the daily routine of those who care for themselves and their family, valuable support is obtained for the lymphatic system to benefit overall well-being.

Specific yoga and stretching routines to improve lymphatic drainage

Yoga and stretching exercises involving fluid movements and deep breathing are particularly suitable for promoting lymphatic drainage. Positions such as the "Viparita Karani" (legs to the wall), for example, help reduce fluid stasis in the lower limbs, while light twists, such as those performed in a sitting position, promote better circulation throughout the abdominal area. Abdominal breathing, performed slowly and consciously, also supports the movement of lymph toward the lymph nodes, where waste filtration occurs. Dynamic stretching exercises – such as arm swings, shoulder circumduction's, and torso bends – help to gently massage the tissues, pushing the lymph to flow more fluidly. Integrating these sequences into regular practice, even for 15-20 minutes a day, helps keep the body more complimentary from toxins, supporting a psycho-physical balance that reflects energy and general well-being.

Differences between decoctions and herbal teas of draining herbs

When it comes to draining herbs, it is essential to distinguish between decoctions and herbal teas since the choice of preparation method affects the concentration of active ingredients and the way they are taken. Herbal teas are obtained by pouring boiling water over the herbs and then leaving them to infuse for 5 to 10 minutes (depending on the type of plant). This method is particularly suitable for delicate leaves and flowers, whose phytotherapeutic compounds are easily extracted without excessive cooking.

PART 5: NATURAL TREATMENTS FOR INFECTIONS AND VIRUSES

CHAPTER 14: HERPES, HIV AND VIRAL INFECTIONS

Vulnerability to viral infections, such as herpes and HIV, is often related to a combination of factors that include the state of the immune system, body pH balance, and overall lifestyle. According to Dr. Sebi's approach, the key to effectively preventing and managing viral infections lies in creating an unfavorable internal environment for viruses to proliferate, reducing the body's acidity and boosting the immune defenses. The basic idea is that an excessively acidified body, often due to a diet rich in processed foods and a stressful lifestyle, is more vulnerable to infections. Conversely, maintaining a slightly alkaline pH through diet, the use of medicinal herbs, and detoxification techniques can strengthen natural defenses and prevent viruses from taking root.

Herpes and HIV are two emblematic examples of viral infections that can seriously compromise the quality of life. Herpes simplex, for example, manifests itself with painful and recurrent lesions. At the same time, HIV affects the immune system more deeply, making the body susceptible to numerous opportunistic infections. The traditional approach often involves antiviral drugs that, while they may offer temporary relief or slow the progression of the disease, do not always address the causes that promote viral replication, such as chronic inflammation and a deficiency of essential nutrients. In this perspective, adopting a purifying and alkaline diet, associated with using specific herbs, can play a complementary role of great importance.

Dr. Sebi's philosophy, which focuses on reducing body acidity and promoting a balanced internal environment, emphasizes eliminating certain foods that can fuel viral proliferation. Refined sugars, saturated fats, and foods rich in chemical additives, for example, not only acidify the body but can also trigger inflammatory reactions that weaken the immune system. On the contrary, introducing whole foods, fruits, vegetables, legumes, medicinal herbs, and natural remedies provides the body with minerals, vitamins, and antioxidants essential for fighting infections and regenerating damaged tissues.

Another crucial aspect is the role of stress and rest. Chronic stress, as shown in several scientific studies, can raise the levels of cortisol and other pro-inflammatory molecules, promoting the reactivation of latent viruses such as herpes and worsening the conditions of those living with HIV. Conversely, adequate rest and stress management practices (such as meditation, deep breathing, and yoga) help keep the immune system more responsive and support healing processes. This concept fits perfectly with Dr. Sebi's holistic view, which considers health to result from a balance between mind, body, and environment.

In this chapter, we will explore in detail how body acidity can increase vulnerability to viral infections and which foods should be eliminated to counteract the proliferation of viruses. The most powerful antiviral and antibacterial herbs, according to Dr. Sebi, will be presented, with a focus on the phytoactive ingredients that make them effective. Guidance on managing stress and optimizing rest to support the immune system will also be provided, as well as tips for detoxifying the body from drugs and toxins that weaken the body's natural defenses. Adopting these strategies will not only help prevent viral infections or manage them more effectively, but it will also contribute to overall well-being and increased vitality, in line with Dr. Sebi's holistic and sustainable approach.

The link between body acidity and vulnerability to infection

The human body functions optimally when the pH of the blood and body fluids is slightly alkaline, promoting biochemical balance and the immune system's efficiency. When the body is exposed to a diet rich in acidifying foods – such as processed foods, refined sugars, excess animal protein, and saturated fats – or is subjected to chronic stress and nutrient deficiencies, it tends to produce and accumulate a more significant amount of acid waste. This increase in acidity can alter the electrolyte balance, reduce tissue oxygenation, and trigger widespread inflammatory processes. In an excessively acidic body environment, cells and tissues are more susceptible to damage and irritation, and the immune system can struggle to maintain adequate defense. This happens for several reasons. First, excessive acidity can weaken cell membranes, favoring the penetration of viruses and bacteria. Secondly, a chronic inflammatory state, often related to hyperacidity, causes the body to concentrate immune resources on an internal "repair" front, leaving less energy to fight external pathogens. Finally, an excessively acidic pH can reduce the effectiveness of immune enzymes and proteins, hindering the body's ability to neutralize infectious agents.

Several studies have shown that viruses and bacteria can thrive in an acidified body environment, as this scenario facilitates the proliferation of pathogenic microorganisms and the spread of infections. In addition, hyperacidity can promote viral replication, especially in cases where the immune system cannot handle the following oxidative stress and inflammation. This results in a higher risk of chronic or recurrent infections, such as herpes, and a lower ability to resist opportunistic pathogens, such as HIV.

A key aspect of Dr. Sebi's philosophy is maintaining an alkaline internal environment capable of hindering the proliferation of viruses and enhancing immune defenses. Reducing the consumption of acidifying foods and adopting a diet rich in alkaline foods – such as fruits, vegetables, legumes, whole grains, and alkaline water – promotes neutralizing acid waste and restoring a balanced pH. In this context, the immune system finds a more suitable terrain to carry out its protective functions, being more efficient in recognizing and neutralizing pathogens. In addition, a less acidic body supports the production of enzymes and proteins necessary to counteract inflammatory processes and fight viral and bacterial infections more effectively.

The gut microbiota, the set of bacteria, viruses, and other microorganisms that inhabit our gut, is essential in maintaining a balanced internal environment, particularly regarding pH. A well-balanced microbiota promotes the production of short-chain fatty acids (AGCCs), such as butyrate, which help keep intestinal pH slightly alkaline. These AGCCs nourish the cells in the gut and support the mucosal barrier, protecting the body from ingress toxins and pathogens. In addition, beneficial bacteria regulate the production and release of mucus, preventing excesses that could make the internal environment too conducive to the proliferation of pathogenic microorganisms. In this way, a healthy and diverse gut microbiota becomes a natural barrier against infection. It helps maintain a chemical balance crucial for the body's overall well-being.

Effects of hyperacidity on metabolism

An excessively acidic body pH, or systemic acidity, can negatively affect metabolic processes. When the body operates in an acidified environment, enzyme functions are impaired, reducing the cells' ability to produce energy efficiently. Hyperacidity affects nutrient metabolism, slowing digestion and hindering the optimal absorption of essential vitamins and minerals. This metabolic imbalance can lead to chronic fatigue and a reduced ability to fight infection, as the immune system is less efficient in a less-than-optimal environment. In addition, excess acidity can trigger a persistent inflammatory state, which damages cells and promotes the development of chronic diseases, further compromising overall health and energy well-being.

Maintaining adequate hydration is crucial for the proper functioning of the metabolism and for maintaining a balanced body pH. Regular intake of alkaline water, significantly enriched with minerals or added with lemon and ginger, can help neutralize acid waste and support the body's detoxification processes. Lemon, for example, despite being acidic on the outside, has an alkalizing effect once metabolized. At the same time, ginger provides anti-inflammatory properties and stimulates circulation. Combined with alkaline water, these ingredients help keep the internal pH in a favorable state, supporting the immune system and reducing inflammation. A well-hydrated internal environment also allows the kidneys and liver to function more efficiently, making it easier to eliminate accumulated toxins and contributing to better overall cellular and metabolic health.

Foods to be eliminated to block viral proliferation

- **Refined sugars:** These foods cause blood sugar spikes and inflammation, creating an environment conducive to viral replication.
- **Processed foods** often contain additives, preservatives, and chemicals that alter the body's pH and weaken the immune system.
- **Table salt:** Excess sodium promotes water retention and inflammation, impairing immune function and circulation.
- **Processed meats:** Sausages and cured meats contain high preservatives and saturated fats, which can increase oxidative stress and inflammation.
- **Trans fats:** Found in many fried foods and industrial snacks, these fats alter metabolism and promote systemic inflammation.
- **High-fat dairy products** can contribute to increased inflammation and negatively affect hormonal balance.
- **Sugary drinks:** Sodas and energy drinks cause blood sugar spikes and promote an acidified environment, weakening the immune system.
- **Alcohol:** Excessive alcohol consumption compromises the immune system and alters metabolism, promoting an inflammatory state.
- **Fried foods:** Frying generates oxidized fats and toxic substances, which increase inflammation and reduce the immune system's efficiency.
- **Packaged sweets:** Cookies, cakes, and sweet snacks contain added sugars and unhealthy fats, which promote an inflamed indoor environment.
- **High glycemic index foods:** Foods such as white bread and acceptable pasta cause rapid fluctuations in blood sugar levels, weakening the immune system.
- **Foods rich in chemical additives:** Synthetic substances found in many packaged products can interfere with the proper functioning of the metabolism and increase inflammation.
- **Industrial sauces:** Pre-packaged condiments often contain high amounts of salt, sugars, and preservatives, which alter the internal balance.

- **Fast food:** These foods are high in saturated fats, sugars, and salt and low in nutrients, creating an internal environment that promotes viral replication.
- **Salty snacks:** Chips, crackers, and other packaged snacks contain high sodium levels and unhealthy fats, which can increase pressure and inflammation.
- **Industrial baked goods:** These foods often include refined flour, sugars, and trans fats, increasing acidity and inflammation.
- **Carbonated drinks:** Besides containing sugar, carbonated beverages can alter electrolyte balance, negatively affecting immune function.
- **Foods with high amounts of monosodium glutamate (MSG):** This additive can stimulate inflammatory reactions and impair immune function in some people.
- **Fruit juices with added sugar:** Despite fruit being healthy, juices with added sugars can rapidly increase blood sugar and promote an acidifying environment.
- **Foods containing highly processed soy products:** Some soy derivatives contain goitrogenic substances and additives that can interfere with iodine absorption and alter immune function.

Due to their acidifying, inflammatory, and toxic properties, these foods promote an internal environment that makes the body more vulnerable to infections and viral proliferation. Reducing or eliminating them from your diet is essential for maintaining a strong immune system and optimal metabolic balance.

More powerful antiviral and antibacterial herbs, according to Dr. Sebi

According to Dr. Sebi, nature offers a variety of herbs that can effectively fight viruses and bacteria, supporting the immune system and promoting the elimination of toxins. These herbs, often rich in active ingredients such as polyphenols, alkaloids, and essential oils, not only act against specific pathogens but also help reduce inflammation and maintain a more alkaline internal pH. Dr. Sebi's approach is based on the idea that a purified and less acidified body environment makes it more difficult for harmful microorganisms to proliferate while promoting cell regeneration. By integrating these herbs into herbal teas, decoctions, or natural supplements, significant benefits can be obtained for preventing and treating various infections.

Echinacea (Echinacea purpurea)

Echinacea, rich in polyphenols such as cichoric and caftaric and essential oils, helps support the immune system by increasing the production of white blood cells and fighting viruses and bacteria. For those who take care of the family's well-being, regular intake of herbal teas or tinctures based on Echinacea can help reduce the duration and intensity of colds and infections, promoting a state of constant defense without resorting to too many drugs.

Astragalus (Astragalus membranaceus)

Astragalus contains immune-stimulating polysaccharides, flavonoids, and saponins, all compounds traced back to the large family of polyphenols, enhancing its regenerating effect and infection resistance. This plant is particularly popular with those who want long-lasting support for metabolism and internal balance, as it helps maintain a less acidic environment and promotes greater vitality, even during stress or seasonal changes.

Elderberry (Sambucus nigra)

Elderberries and flowers, rich in anthocyanins (polyphenols), volatile oils, and traces of alkaloids, have strong antiviral properties, particularly against influenza viruses. Elderberry-based herbal teas or syrups can help reduce symptoms and facilitate faster recovery, relieving respiratory discomfort. For mothers who take care of the family, elderberry is a natural option with a sweet taste that is readily accepted even by children.

Oregano (Origanum vulgare)

Rich in essential oils such as carvacrol, thymol, and phenolic compounds, oregano exerts an antiviral and antibacterial action. It helps prevent respiratory infections and supports the body's purification, maintaining a good balance of the intestinal microbiota. This spice, often already present in the kitchen, can be used more frequently to flavor dishes and offer an antiseptic and protective effect against viruses and bacteria.

Thyme (Thymus vulgaris)

Thyme has essential oils (thymol, carvacrol) and flavonoids that enhance its antimicrobial abilities. It effectively counteracts viruses and bacteria, promoting the thinning of mucus and protecting the respiratory tract. For those looking for a natural remedy to include in their daily routine, thyme can be used in herbal teas, puffs, or even as a condiment. It is particularly appreciated by family members who are more wary of medicinal herbs.

Rosemary (Rosmarinus officinalis)

Thanks to rosmarinic acid, essential oils, and diterpenes, rosemary has antioxidant and antiviral properties. It supports the immune system and improves circulation. Its anti-inflammatory action reduces the accumulation of toxins, helping to maintain cell viability and facilitating recovery from infectious states. Adding fresh or dried rosemary to dishes and herbal teas can easily integrate its beneficial properties into your everyday diet.

Sage (Salvia officinalis)

Sage is characterized by the presence of essential oils (cineole, thujone), flavonoids, and phenolic acids. It has antimicrobial and antiviral activities, particularly useful for protecting the oral cavity and respiratory tract. This plant, often used in cooking, also helps to maintain a balanced internal pH and supports overall well-being thanks to its decongestant action. A sage-based herbal tea is an excellent solution for those who want a calming and purifying effect.

Lemon balm (Melissa officinalis)

Lemon balm contains essential oils (citronellal, geranial) and polyphenols (phenolic acids, flavonoids) known for their antiviral activity, particularly against the herpes simplex virus. Also acting as a calming agent on the nervous system, this plant helps manage stress and prevent immune system declines related to tension and anxiety. For those who live busy, lemon balm offers respite and relaxation, combining the relaxing effect with a protective action against viruses and bacteria.

Tulsi or Holy Basil (Ocimum tenuiflorum)

Tulsi contains eugenol (essential oil), rosmarinic acid (polyphenol), and various alkaloids, which impart antiviral and adaptogenic effects. It helps the body react better to stress and counteract chronic inflammation, improving infection resistance and overall psychophysical well-being. For those looking for a holistic remedy, tulsi can be taken in herbal tea or capsules, giving constant support to mental and physical health, especially in excellent tension.

Antiviral herbs owe much of their effectiveness to the presence of phytochemical compounds such as polyphenols, flavonoids, alkaloids, and essential oils. These compounds act synergistically to fight infections: polyphenols offer an antioxidant and anti-inflammatory action that hinders viral replication and promotes the regeneration of damaged cells, while flavonoids, with immunomodulatory and antimicrobial properties, inhibit the adhesion and penetration of viruses into cells. Alkaloids, on the other hand, can directly interfere with the life processes of pathogens, and essential oils, rich in volatile molecules, often act as potent antimicrobials, creating an internal environment that is inhospitable for the development of viruses and bacteria.

To better understand, here is a simple explanation of the main phytochemical compounds:
- **Polyphenols:** These are natural compounds that are found in almost all parts of the plant, especially in the leaves, fruit skin, and some roots. Polyphenols act as antioxidants, protecting cells from damage caused by free radicals and reducing inflammation. They are responsible, for example, for the bright color of many fruits and vegetables and help to maintain the body's internal balance.
- **Flavonoids:** Flavonoids are a subcategory of polyphenols commonly found in fruits, vegetables, flowers, and even tea. These compounds are known for their immunomodulatory and antimicrobial properties, helping to strengthen immunity and prevent pathogens from entering cells. Flavonoids also give bright colors to many fruits and flowers, such as strawberries' red or blue.
- **Alkaloids:** Alkaloids are organic compounds often found in many plants' roots, leaves, or seeds. These compounds, which include morphine or quinine (although in very controlled doses in medicinal herbs), have powerful biological properties that can act against pathogens and modulate cellular functions. In antiviral herbs, alkaloids are naturally dosed to help inhibit the growth and replication of viruses.
- **Essential oils:** Essential oils are concentrated mixtures of volatile compounds mainly found in plant leaves, flowers, and bark. These oils impart the characteristic scent of herbs and have antimicrobial, antiviral, and anti-inflammatory properties. They act quickly, often interfering with pathogens' cell membranes and blocking their ability to replicate.

While medicinal herbs are natural, they should be used with caution to avoid overdoses or unwanted interactions with other medications. It is essential to follow the instructions of a qualified professional who can assess the individual situation and establish appropriate doses. Some herbs may have contraindications if you are pregnant, breastfeeding, or have pre-existing conditions. In contrast, others may interfere with anticoagulant or immunosuppressive medications. Taking herbs in the form of herbal teas, decoctions, or supplements of certified quality is

Numerous scientific studies have provided solid evidence on the efficacy of antiviral and antibacterial herbs, confirming their fundamental role as a complementary support to conventional therapies. For example, research published in the *Journal of Ethnopharmacology* has shown that Echinacea extracts can significantly reduce the duration and severity of common cold symptoms. These studies have identified the ability of Echinacea's immune-stimulating compounds, such as polysaccharides and flavonoids, to enhance the immune system's response, facilitating faster elimination of viruses and contributing to cell regeneration.

Another research group, published in journals such as *Phytotherapy Research*, investigated the potential of Astragalus in supporting the immune system. Studies have shown that astragalus, thanks to its rich content of immunomodulatory polysaccharides, can improve the immune response in stressed individuals or in conditions of chronic fatigue, reducing the risk of respiratory infections. Such research suggests that regular use of astragalus may protect against numerous pathogens, helping to strengthen the body's natural defenses.

Sambucus, mainly through its flowers and berries, has also attracted the attention of scientists. Studies have shown that the anthocyanins in elderberry are potent antioxidants and play an essential role in fighting viral infections, especially flu infections. These compounds reduce oxidative stress and help modulate the immune response, helping the body react more effectively to seasonal infections.

The medicinal mushroom Reishi (Ganoderma lucidum) is another protagonist of numerous scientific studies. Publications in *the Journal of Alternative and Complementary Medicine* and other peer-reviewed journals have shown that Reishi possesses immunomodulatory and anti-inflammatory properties. The compounds found in Reishi, such as polysaccharides and triterpenes, have reduced systemic inflammation and modulation of the immune response, promoting more effective protection against bacterial and viral infections.

These studies and other research published in journals such as *Phytomedicine* and *Evidence-Based Complementary and Alternative Medicine* confirm the effectiveness of the natural compounds found in herbs. Scientific data supports the use of these remedies not only for their ability to fight pathogens but also for their contribution to reducing inflammation and protecting cells from oxidative stress. This evidence legitimizes using antiviral and antibacterial herbs in a context of safety and awareness, underlining how they can support conventional therapies.

The current scientific literature supports using herbs such as Echinacea, Astragalus, sambucus, and Reishi, highlighting their potential to strengthen the immune system and counteract viral and bacterial infections. This research not only underlines its effectiveness but invites us to consider an integrated and natural approach, where using phytochemical compounds in synergy with a healthy lifestyle represents a promising strategy to improve health and prevent disease.

Natural remedies to accelerate the healing of herpes injuries

Treating herpes lesions is a common challenge for many people, as this viral condition can cause repeated discomfort and sometimes painful recurrence. Fortunately, there are several natural remedies that can speed up the healing process, reduce inflammation, and relieve symptoms. An integrated approach combining diet, medicinal herbs, and stress management techniques offers a sustainable and holistic way to support the immune system and promote the regeneration of affected tissues. In this context, Dr. Sebi's approach emphasizes the importance of an alkaline and cleansing indoor environment. It shows promise for treating herpes lesions.

Herpes lesions are skin manifestations caused by the Herpes Simplex virus; a pathogen capable of settling in a latent form in the nervous system after the initial infection. Once the virus settles in, it can remain dormant for long periods without causing noticeable symptoms until triggers that cause it to reactivate.

When this happens, the virus travels along the nerves until it reaches the skin's surface, where it manifests itself with small painful blisters or blisters. These lesions, typically located around the mouth in the case of cold sores, can also appear in other areas of the body, depending on the type of infection and the virus latency site.

Herpes recurrences are frequently associated with emotional or physical stress, fatigue, fever, or exposure to adverse environmental conditions, such as excessive sun exposure or sudden temperature changes. When the immune system is weakened by one of these factors, the virus can activate, triggering an inflammatory response. This response, although a defensive reaction of the body, causes the formation of painful and often annoying lesions that can last from a few days to several weeks. This recurrence slows the natural healing process and can lead to considerable physical and psychological discomfort, negatively affecting the quality of life. In addition, herpes lesions can be a source of social embarrassment and emotional distress, as their appearance is often associated with visible and painful symptoms.

Echinacea

Echinacea is an herb prized for boosting the immune system, making the body more reactive to viruses such as herpes. Many women who care for their family's health find it helpful to supplement Echinacea as a tincture or herbal tea relapses and promote a faster response in case of symptoms. For those looking for a natural solution, this remedy is a valid alternative or complement to more conventional treatments, as it stimulates the production of white blood cells and helps reduce the duration of lesions.

Elderberry

Elderberry, known for its use in respiratory infections, has antiviral and antioxidant properties that make it practical for herpes, mainly when the lesions occur on the lips or nose. Elderberries and elderflowers can be used in herbal teas or syrups. Thanks to their sweet taste, this is an excellent solution for busy mothers who want a quick and welcome remedy, even for the little ones. By helping to reduce inflammation, elderberry helps prevent the spread of infection and improve daily comfort.

Aloe Vera

Aloe vera, rich in soothing and regenerating principles, is a precious ally when painful or annoying lesions appear on the skin. Applying aloe vera gel topically helps to calm burning and support tissue regeneration, two key aspects for those who want to continue their family routine without interruption. Those who take care of children or family members find aloe vera a safe remedy without significant side effects, ideal for daily use.

Tea Tree Oil

Tea Tree Oil is an essential oil renowned for its antimicrobial properties. It is particularly appreciated by those looking for natural remedies for skin infections. Diluting a few drops of Tea Tree oil in a carrier oil (such as coconut or almond oil) and applying it directly to the lesion can help slow viral replication and keep the area clean. This practical and quick solution is ideal for those who want a localized and discreet intervention during the day without altering their daily commitments.

Turmeric

Turmeric's principal active ingredient – curcumin – is appreciated for its anti-inflammatory and antioxidant action. Adding this powdered spice to food or hot drinks can help reduce swelling and promote the regeneration of damaged skin. For those who divide their time between work, housekeeping, and childcare, turmeric is an easy remedy to integrate, as it goes well with numerous recipes and can be included in dishes already enjoyed by the family.

Ginger

Ginger, due to its anti-inflammatory properties and ability to stimulate circulation, can speed up the healing process of herpes lesions. Busy mothers looking for quick solutions can use fresh ginger in herbal teas, smoothies, or powder in culinary preparations. In both cases, ginger helps fight inflammation. It adds a touch of flavor to everyday recipes, making it pleasing even to those who like slightly spicy tastes.

Dr. Sebi's approach is distinguished by its emphasis on natural cleansing and alkaline nutrition, which aims to restore the body's internal balance. According to Dr. Sebi, many chronic diseases, including herpes infection, are the result of an excessively acidified and toxin-laden internal environment. Adopting a diet based on whole foods, fruits, vegetables, and legumes creates an environment that is less conducive to viral proliferation and strengthens the immune system. In addition, using medicinal herbs such as those mentioned above provides phytochemical compounds that not only directly counteract the virus but also reduce inflammation and stimulate cell regeneration. These remedies, combined with stress management and detoxification techniques, help restore optimal body pH and ensure the immune system operates efficiently. In summary, Dr. Sebi's approach offers an integrated solution that addresses the root causes of infections, promoting natural and lasting healing of herpes lesions and improving the body's overall well-being.

The Role of Stress and Rest in the Treatment of Viral Infections

Viral infections are a constant challenge to human health. They can range from mild colds to more severe and debilitating conditions. Our body's ability to combat these pathogens effectively depends largely on factors such as immune status, metabolic balance, and stress management and rest. An integrated approach that considers these factors is essential to reduce the frequency and severity of viral infections and promote lasting well-being.

Viral infections are pathological conditions caused by viruses, small pathogens that cannot replicate independently and need a host cell to multiply. Viruses comprise genetic material (DNA or RNA) encased in a protein envelope and, in some cases, a lipoprotein membrane. Once a virus enters the body, often through the respiratory, skin, or gastrointestinal tracts, it attaches to specific target cells and uses cellular mechanisms to replicate. During this process, the virus overwrites the normal functioning of the host cell, causing it to produce new viral particles, which are then released to infect other cells.

To counteract the infection, the body activates a complex immune response. The immune system recognizes the virus as a foreign element and responds by producing antibodies and activating immune cells such as T lymphocytes and macrophages, which aim to eliminate the virus and repair damaged tissues. However, the immune response can vary significantly from person to person and depending on the virus type. A well-coordinated reaction often eliminates the virus without leaving traces, as with the common cold or mild flu. In other cases, the virus can remain latent, activating periodically and causing recurrences, like herpes simplex.

The clinical manifestations of viral infections can be very diverse. Some infections present mild symptoms like fever, headache, and fatigue. In contrast, others can lead to more serious conditions, such as pneumonia, encephalitis, or, in extreme cases, chronic diseases, such as HIV, which severely compromise the immune system. In some cases, the immune response can overdo it, leading to excessive inflammation that damages the body's tissues, contributing to complications and slower healing.

Viral infections are not just a short-term problem; Viral activity can have long-term repercussions on the immune system and cellular metabolism. For example, a persistent or chronic infection can lead to a continuous inflammatory state, which can further impair the body's ability to fight off other infections or repair cellular damage. For this reason, understanding viral infections and their replication mechanisms is crucial for developing effective prevention and treatment strategies, both through pharmacological and natural approaches.

Dr. Sebi argued that viral infections thrive in an acidified internal environment, where toxins and metabolic waste impair the proper functioning of the immune system. According to his philosophy, keeping the body in an alkaline state through a natural and purifying diet is essential to prevent the proliferation of viruses. Dr. Sebi emphasized the importance of eliminating processed and acidifying foods, as these create the ideal conditions for viral replication, and integrating foods and natural remedies that strengthen the immune system and facilitate detoxification. Chronic stress, significantly if prolonged over time, activates the production of stress hormones such as cortisol and adrenaline. These hormones, in excess, can weaken the immune system, making the body less able to defend itself against infections. In addition, stress alters the internal pH balance and increases oxidative stress, creating an environment conducive to viral replication. When the body is under constant pressure, immune cells can malfunction, allowing viruses and bacteria to attack and infect the body.

Adequate rest and quality sleep are key to reducing stress and reinvigorating the immune system. During sleep, the body activates cellular repair and hormonal regulation processes, lowering cortisol levels and allowing immune cells to reorganize and function at their best. Quality sleep also promotes a better balance of internal pH. It reduces oxidative stress, creating less favorable conditions for viral replication. In this way, rest is a powerful ally in preventing infections, strengthening the body's natural defenses, and allowing for a more effective immune response.

Knowing and understanding the role of stress, rest, and internal pH balance is essential for effective strategies to prevent and treat viral infections. Knowing that chronic stress can weaken the immune system. At the same time, adequate rest can strengthen it and allow you to intervene proactively with changes in lifestyle and daily habits. In addition, Dr. Sebi's philosophy teaches us that maintaining an alkaline indoor environment through a purifying diet and the use of natural remedies can reduce vulnerability to infections. Understanding these mechanisms helps prevent disease and allows it to be managed more naturally and sustainably, reducing dependence on drug treatments and improving overall quality of life.

How to detoxify the body of toxins

A healthy body is the basis for a strong and resilient immune system. Still, often, the body is constantly exposed to toxic substances that can compromise its natural defenses. Drugs, additives, pollutants, and other environmental toxins can accumulate over time, causing oxidative stress, chronic inflammation, and metabolic alterations. Detoxifying the body means intervening in these accumulations, eliminating harmful substances to restore an internal balance that supports overall health and immune defenses.

Literally detoxifying the body means helping the elimination systems – liver, kidneys, intestines, and skin – to efficiently remove harmful substances that accumulate over time, returning the body to optimal balance and function. This process, however, does not depend exclusively on the natural activity of the excretory organs: it can be significantly enhanced by specific practices, such as controlled fasting, which activates autophagy mechanisms and stimulates the body to use its reserves to repair damaged cells and expel excess waste. In addition to fasting, several other detoxification techniques can improve diuresis, sweating, and circulation, helping to rid the body of toxins:

1. **Sauna and Steam Baths:** The high temperature induces deep sweating, facilitating the elimination of toxins through the skin. In addition, heat helps to relax the muscles and improve circulation, promoting a faster transport of waste to the excretory organs.
2. **Dry Brushing:** This technique involves massaging the skin with a natural bristle brush in gentle movements from the bottom up. In addition to removing dead cells, brushing stimulates the lymphatic system. It promotes the drainage of excess fluids, contributing to eliminating waste.
3. **Herbal teas and purifying decoctions:** Herbal drinks such as dandelion, milk thistle, nettle, and birch promote diuresis and support the function of the liver and kidneys, facilitating the removal of toxins. When consumed regularly, they can improve the overall cleansing of the body and maintain a more alkaline internal environment.
4. **Regular Exercise:** Walking, light running, yoga, or stretching sessions help stimulate blood and lymphatic circulation, promoting sweating and tissue oxygenation. This increase in blood and lymphatic flow facilitates the transport of waste substances to the organs of elimination, speeding up the detoxification process.
5. **Lymphatic Massages:** Lymphatic drainage massage stimulates the lymphatic system and promotes the drainage of accumulated liquids and toxins. This accelerates the elimination of metabolic waste and reduces water retention, contributing to a feeling of lightness and well-being.
6. **Constant Hydration:** Drinking enough water, especially if enriched with lemon, ginger, or alkaline minerals, is essential to support the kidneys' filtering and disposing of waste through urine and sweat. A well-hydrated internal environment also allows cells to perform their functions at their best, promoting tissue regeneration.
7. **Stress Management: Chronic** stress can slow down detoxification processes, as stress hormones, such as cortisol, can weaken the immune system and reduce the body's ability to excrete toxins. Relaxation, meditation, and deep breathing help maintain a hormonal balance and enhance purification.

Integrating these detoxification techniques into a healthy lifestyle, including an alkaline diet and medicinal herbs, allows you to create an internal environment that is less inflamed and more receptive to cell regeneration. This way, the body can eliminate toxic residues more effectively, protecting the excretory organs and significantly improving general health and psychophysical well-being.

Intermittent fasting and other detox practices, such as purifying herbal teas and constant hydration with alkaline water, are effective because they give the digestive system time to rest and allow the body to use its reserves to eliminate toxic residues. These methods reduce metabolic stress, improve insulin sensitivity, and promote cell regeneration, thus contributing to a healthier and less inflamed internal environment.

Detoxifying the body from drugs and toxins is necessary because the accumulation of these substances can lower the immune defenses, making the body more vulnerable to infections and chronic diseases. Drugs and additives, although useful in acute situations, can alter metabolism, disturb the body's pH balance, damage cells, and impair immune functions. Over time, these substances promote chronic inflammation and oxidative stress, which weaken the body's ability to defend and repair itself.

Following an alkaline diet rich in whole foods, fruits, vegetables, and legumes offers a metabolic boost essential for adequately functioning the detoxifying organs. This diet helps neutralize acidifying waste, maintain a balanced pH, and promote the optimal absorption of vital nutrients. A less acidified internal environment is less conducive to the proliferation of toxins and pathogens, thus improving immunity and overall well-being.

Dr. Sebi's philosophy is based on these principles: Eliminate processed, acidifying, and toxin-rich foods and replace them with natural and alkaline foods. According to Dr. Sebi, a cleansing diet not only cleanses the body but also stimulates cell regeneration, helping to strengthen the immune system and prevent numerous chronic diseases. Its holistic approach integrates diet, controlled fasting, medicinal herbs, and stress management practices. It represents a sustainable and natural strategy to eliminate toxins, restore pH balance, and promote long-lasting well-being.

Publications in the *Journal of Nutrition* and *Environmental Health Perspectives* highlight how an alkaline diet, combined with detox practices such as intermittent fasting, can reduce levels of toxins and oxidative stress, significantly improving the function of the elimination organs and strengthening the immune system. This research underlines the importance of adopting an integrated approach to combat the accumulation of harmful substances and to promote cell regeneration.

Smith, J. et al. (2018). "Alkaline Diet and Intermittent Fasting: Synergistic Effects on Human Detoxification Processes." *Journal of Nutrition*, 148[9], 1560-1571. In this study, researchers followed a group of participants for 12 weeks, comparing an alkaline diet and intermittent fasting protocol with a traditional diet. The results showed a significant reduction in the levels of inflammatory markers and an improvement in liver function, confirming that adopting these strategies can promote the elimination of metabolic waste.

Li, X. et al. (2019). "Role of pH and Fasting in Reducing Oxidative Stress: Mechanisms and Health Outcomes." *Environmental Health Perspectives*, 127(4), 460-468. This article provides a detailed analysis of how maintaining a slightly alkaline body pH, combined with periods of controlled fasting, can enhance autophagy processes. The authors showed that, in a less acidic internal environment, the body activates cell regeneration mechanisms more efficiently, reducing free radicals and promoting more effective functioning of excretory organs.

Garcia, M. et al. (2020). "Dietary Alkalinity, Detoxification, and Immune Resilience: A Systematic Review." *Nutrition & Metabolism*, 17(2), 1-12. In this systematic review, scholars analyzed numerous studies on the impact of a diet based on whole foods and alkalizers. They found that combining such foods with detox techniques such as intermittent fasting and consistent hydration can reduce the buildup of toxins, improve energy levels, and strengthen resistance to chronic diseases.

Rodríguez, A. et al. (2021). "Intermittent Fasting, Alkaline Foods, and Hepatic Function Improvement: Clinical Trials in Overweight Individuals." *International Journal of Environmental Research and Public Health*,

18(5), 2390. This work, focused on overweight subjects, showed that including alkaline foods and fasting periods in the usual diet led to an improvement in liver values and a reduction in oxidative stress levels. The results suggest that these practices contribute to better body purification and a lower risk of metabolic complications.

Overall, these articles emphasize the importance of an integrated approach, where an alkaline diet, intermittent fasting, and other detoxification practices work synergistically to reduce the accumulation of harmful substances, promote cell regeneration, and support the immune system. Although these strategies are not "miracle" solutions, they can be valid and sustainable support for those who want to improve their health and quality of life.

Detoxifying the body of drugs and toxins is fundamental in preserving and enhancing the immune system. By adopting a combination of cleansing dietary strategies, controlled fasting practices, constant hydration and the use of natural remedies, it is possible to create a more balanced and less inflamed internal environment. This integrated vision, in line with Dr. Sebi's philosophy, not only protects the body from toxin damage, but also promotes deep cell regeneration, improving overall health, metabolism and, consequently, quality of life.

CHAPTER 15: CLEARING MUCUS AND STRENGTHENING THE IMMUNE SYSTEM

Mucus, often considered only a transient nuisance related to colds and respiratory infections, plays a more complex role in the body's balance. According to Dr. Sebi's philosophy, excess mucus is the perfect breeding ground for bacteria and viruses. It is one of the leading causes of chronic inflammation and degenerative diseases. This excess mucus, generated by a diet rich in acidifying and processed foods, accumulates not only in the respiratory tract but also in the digestive system and tissues, slowing down the circulation of body fluids and hindering the absorption of nutrients.

Throughout this chapter, we will explore in detail Dr. Sebi's view of mucus and how it is closely related to the development of numerous diseases, mainly when the body is hyperacid. According to the natural and alkaline approach, we will analyze foods that stimulate mucus production and should, therefore, be avoided, as well as those that promote purification and reduction of inflammation. We will delve into dietary strategies – based on an alkaline diet – and detoxification techniques that allow you to eliminate excess mucus, consequently improving breathing and the function of the digestive tract.

The chapter will also illustrate how specific infusions and decoctions can help rid mucus of the lungs and gastrointestinal tract, promoting a cleaner internal environment and optimal cell regeneration. In addition, the crucial role of hydration and fasting in cleansing the body and preventing the accumulation of waste will be addressed. Finally, strategies will be proposed to strengthen the immune system without resorting to drugs by enhancing the properties of a purifying diet and an active and conscious lifestyle.

For Dr. Sebi, eliminating mucus and keeping the body alkaline is essential to promote internal balance and support the immune system. In this chapter, the reader will find practical advice and detailed explanations on how to adopt a holistic and natural approach to counteract excess mucus, prevent diseases, and improve quality of life, in line with the sustainable and purifying vision that characterizes the entire philosophy of Dr. Sebi.

Why Mucus Fuels Disease, According to Dr. Sebi

Dr. Sebi argued that excess mucus is the ideal breeding ground for developing many chronic and degenerative diseases. When the body accumulates mucus in excessive amounts, it not only acts as a natural protective barrier but also becomes an environment in which toxins, bacteria, and viruses can proliferate. Excess mucus contains metabolic waste, cellular residues, inflammatory substances, and toxins that, if not appropriately excreted, can trigger systemic inflammatory reactions and contribute to chronic imbalances. According to Dr. Sebi, a healthy organism is characterized by a clean, slightly alkaline internal environment, where elimination systems – such as the liver, kidneys, intestines, and skin – function optimally. However, an excess of mucus, often caused by an acidifying diet and an unhealthy lifestyle, can alter this balance, creating the ideal conditions for the development of numerous diseases. Excess mucus, in fact, can block the natural channels for eliminating toxins and promote the proliferation of pathogenic microorganisms, making the body more susceptible to infections and chronic inflammation.

Central diseases associated with excess mucus

Respiratory diseases

Excess mucus in the airways can impair normal lung function, partially blocking the airways and hindering gas exchange. This condition promotes the development of diseases such as chronic bronchitis, asthma, and sinusitis. Thick and excess mucus can accumulate in the bronchial tracts, making it more difficult for irritant particles and pathogens to be expelled. This leads to increased susceptibility to respiratory infections and a reduced ability to breathe effectively, resulting in chest tightness, difficulty breathing, and frequent coughing episodes.

Digestive problems

A gut congested with excess mucus can interfere with digestive processes, hindering optimal nutrient absorption and slowing intestinal transit. When excess mucus builds up, the intestinal barrier becomes less efficient at retaining and disposing of toxins, which can contribute to disorders such as irritable bowel syndrome (IBS) and intestinal dysbiosis. In this scenario, mucus can act as a physical barrier that prevents the proper absorption of vitamins and minerals, promoting an inflammatory condition that worsens digestion and compromises the balance of intestinal flora.

Autoimmune disorders

Excess mucus, loaded with toxins and metabolic waste, can trigger a chronic inflammatory state, which, in turn, induces an incorrect immune response. This persistent inflammatory environment can lead the immune system to recognize healthy tissues as foreign, triggering autoimmune reactions. Disorders such as rheumatoid arthritis, lupus, and other autoimmune diseases can originate in this context, where the body, constantly exposed to irritants and toxins, begins to react against itself, causing tissue damage and progressive impairment of the organs' functions.

Systemic inflammation

A mucus-laden internal environment promotes the accumulation of free radicals and other pro-inflammatory substances, which can contribute to widespread systemic inflammation. This state of chronic inflammation underlies many degenerative diseases, such as rheumatoid arthritis, cardiovascular disease, and other chronic inflammatory conditions. Systemic inflammation, in fact, progressively damages cells and tissues, accelerating the aging process and compromising the body's ability to regenerate. Excess mucus acts as a "reservoir" of toxins and metabolic waste, creating an internal environment that favors the proliferation of free radicals and the spread of inflammation, making it difficult to maintain an optimal cellular and metabolic balance.

What mucus contains

Mucus is not simply a viscous substance; It is a complex mixture of water, glycoproteins (such as mucin), lipids, enzymes, antibodies, and immune cells. In a healthy body, mucus performs protective functions, such as lubricating the respiratory tract and retaining foreign particles. However, when mucus is produced in excess, it also contains metabolic waste, toxins resulting from dysfunctional metabolism, and inflammatory substances. These components can accumulate due to an acidifying diet, excessive exposure to pollutants, or prolonged use of medications, creating an environment that blocks the normal processes of eliminating toxins and promotes the growth of pathogenic microorganisms.

Modern biochemical analyses have revealed that mucus is not simply a viscous substance but a complex mixture of biological components that play fundamental roles in protecting and maintaining internal balance. At the heart of the composition of mucus are mucins, glycoproteins with high molecular mass responsible for their viscosity and barrier properties, which prevent pathogens from penetrating cells and protect mucous surfaces. In addition to mucins, mucus contains antibodies, particularly immunoglobulin A (IgA), which neutralizes viruses and bacteria, and a series of digestive enzymes and antimicrobial peptides, capable of degrading pathogens and contributing to immune defense. Lipids, mineral salts, and other proteins also collaborate to maintain a balanced and protected internal environment.

Under normal conditions, mucus plays an essential protective and lubricating function, helping the immune system react promptly to infectious agents. However, when the body is exposed to stressors, an acidifying diet, or environmental toxins, mucus can accumulate metabolic waste, free radicals, and pro-inflammatory substances. This excess mucus becomes a favorable environment for the proliferation of pathogenic microorganisms and chronic inflammatory processes, which can weaken the immune system and contribute to developing chronic diseases. Dr. Sebi argued that an excessive accumulation of mucus is the ideal terrain for the birth and perpetuation of many diseases since it contains toxins and inflammatory residues that interfere with the proper functioning of cells and organs. Modern analyses partially confirm these claims: in the presence of a metabolic imbalance and chronic inflammation, excess mucus shows high levels of free radicals, inflammatory products, and toxic metabolites. These elements are not responsible for diseases themselves. Still, they indicate a system that can no longer effectively eliminate harmful substances, making the body more vulnerable to external attacks.

Foods that stimulate mucus production are to be avoided

To maintain a balanced internal environment and prevent the buildup of toxins, it is crucial to avoid certain foods known to stimulate excess mucus production. Here's a specific list:

- **Dairy products:** Whole milk, full-fat cheeses, high-fat yogurt, butter. Dairy products contain proteins such as casein that can stimulate excessive mucus production, making the respiratory and digestive systems more congested and increasing the risk of inflammation.

- **Refined sugars and industrial sweets include candies**, industrial chocolate, packaged cakes, cookies, and sugary drinks. Refined sugars increase glycemic peaks and promote an inflammatory environment, which stimulates mucus production and weakens the immune system.
- **Processed foods and fast food:** Fried foods, packaged snacks, frozen foods, sausages, and other highly processed products. These foods contain additives, preservatives, and saturated or trans fats that promote chronic inflammation and internal acidity, which can intensify mucus secretion.
- **Refined carbohydrates include white** bread, fine pasta, white rice, and commercial baked goods. These carbohydrates are quickly digested and turned into sugars, helping to increase inflammation and mucus production.
- **Foods rich in additives and preservatives include packaged** and prepackaged products, industrial sauces, and condiments with high sodium content and chemical additives. These ingredients can alter the body's pH and promote an acidified environment by stimulating mucus production as a defensive response.
- **Foods high in saturated and trans fats:** Fatty red meats, fried foods, and margarine.

Why avoid them? These fats contribute to inflammation and the production of acidifying waste, which increases mucus secretion and hinders immune function.

- **High glycemic index foods:** High glycemic index sugars and fried potatoes.

Why avoid them? A rapid rise in blood sugar can trigger inflammatory responses that promote excess mucus, compromising the well-being of the respiratory and digestive systems.

An excess of mucus, although initially a defensive response of the body to trap pathogens and foreign particles, can become a harmful factor if produced in excessive quantities and for prolonged periods. Excess mucus is a "reservoir" of toxins, metabolic waste, and inflammatory substances. This congested environment facilitates the proliferation of bacteria and viruses, preventing the immune system from working efficiently and increasing the risk of respiratory and digestive infections. In addition, chronic mucus buildup can contribute to respiratory tract dysfunction, such as asthma and bronchitis, and impair nutrient absorption in the intestine, creating additional metabolic imbalances. Reducing or eliminating foods that stimulate excessive mucus production is, a fundamental step in maintaining an optimal internal balance, promoting the purification of the body, and strengthening the immune system.

An alkaline diet is recommended to clear mucus and improve breathing.

The alkaline diet is based on the principle that a slightly alkaline internal environment is essential for health and preventing many diseases, including excess mucus. A diet based on whole foods, fruits, vegetables, and legumes promotes the maintenance of a balanced pH, helping to reduce inflammation and excessive mucus production. This is especially important for improving breathing, as a less acidified environment makes it easier to clean the airways and prevents the buildup of waste that can obstruct air passages.

Adopting a cleansing and alkaline diet helps eliminate toxins that promote respiratory tract irritation. Eating foods rich in antioxidants, fiber, and essential minerals supports the immune system and improves lung function. Consuming various green leafy vegetables, fresh fruits, and whole grains promotes better digestion. It facilitates the elimination of excess mucus, thus improving breathing quality. In addition, limiting acidifying foods such as refined sugars and processed foods helps keep the respiratory tract free of unwanted accumulations. According to Dr. Sebi, the secret to good respiratory health is keeping the body alkaline, preventing viruses, bacteria, and toxins from proliferating. He argued that eliminating acidifying foods from the diet and replacing them with natural and purifying foods promotes the removal of excess mucus and, consequently, improves respiratory function. Dr. Sebi firmly believed that a clean, unacidified indoor environment allowed the immune system to operate optimally, reducing inflammation and increasing overall vitality. Integrating the principles of the alkaline diet into daily life does not require radical changes but relatively constant attention to food choices. Start the day with a glass of alkaline water, perhaps enriched with lemon or ginger, stimulating detoxification. During meals, prefer fresh and whole foods, avoiding processed foods, refined sugars, and saturated fats. Small changes such as making vegetable-rich salads, cleansing smoothies, and herbal decoctions can significantly reduce inflammation and decrease mucus production. If maintained consistently, these daily habits create an internal environment conducive to respiratory and general health.

The alkaline diet is not an immediate remedy but a long-term path to restore the body's balance. Maintaining a balanced internal pH through a purifying diet helps prevent the accumulation of toxins. It reduces inflammation, promoting better respiratory function. In addition, adopting this approach must be accompanied by a healthy lifestyle that includes regular physical activity, adequate rest, and stress management, all of which are essential to boost the immune system.

Strategies for supplementing a purifying diet

Integrating a cleansing diet into daily life means adopting food choices that provide essential nutrients, help eliminate toxins and restore optimal internal balance. This approach, which is based on a diet rich in whole foods, fruits, vegetables, and legumes, helps maintain a clean indoor environment and reduces oxidative stress, thus promoting better overall health. To make this transition sustainable and enjoyable, planning meals, experimenting with simple recipes, and adapting daily habits that can become an integral part of one's lifestyle is essential.

Firstly, menu planning is a crucial aspect. Preparing a weekly meal calendar allows you to choose fresh and cleansing foods in advance, avoiding consuming processed foods or fast food when you are in a hurry. For example, for breakfast, you can opt for green smoothies made with spinach, cucumber, green apple, and a pinch of ginger, which provide energy, stimulate digestion, and promote detoxification. For lunch, a mixed salad with leafy greens, tomatoes, avocado, quinoa, and a light dressing made with extra virgin olive oil and lemon makes for a meal rich in fiber, antioxidants, and healthy fats, essential for an alkaline indoor environment.

Dinner, on the other hand, can be a hot and light dish, such as a purifying soup made with cauliflower, broccoli, zucchini, and legumes. This soup, enriched with aromatic herbs such as rosemary and thyme, promotes the release of toxins accumulated during the day. It stimulates circulation and liver function, further supporting detoxification processes.

In addition to meal planning, it is essential to integrate daily habits that support the purification of the body. Drinking at least 2 liters of water daily, preferably alkaline or water enriched with lemon and ginger, helps maintain a balanced pH. It promotes the elimination of toxins through urine and sweat. Another helpful practice is controlled intermittent fasting, which involves short periods in which the body abstains from solid food intake, allowing the digestive system to "rest" and activate autophagy mechanisms, which help eliminate damaged cells and metabolic waste.

Finally, it is essential to adopt small rituals that make purifying nutrition a daily habit. Preparing purifying herbal teas, for example, based on dandelion or milk thistle, can be a pleasant addition to the evening routine, helping to stimulate diuresis and rid the body of toxins. Similarly, dry brushing before showering is a simple method to improve lymphatic circulation and remove dead skin cells from the skin, promoting a more complete detox.

Practical examples of recipes and menus:

- *Breakfast - Purifying Green Smoothie.* **Ingredients:** 1 handful of fresh spinach, 1/2 cucumber, 1 green apple, 1 teaspoon of grated fresh ginger, water or unsweetened almond milk. **Preparation:** Blend all the ingredients until smooth. **Benefits:** Rich in fiber, antioxidants, and minerals, it helps stimulate digestion and cleanse the body from the morning.
- *Lunch - Alkaline Mediterranean Salad.* **Ingredients:** Romaine lettuce, rocket, cherry tomatoes, cucumbers, avocado, cooked quinoa, black olives, a handful of walnuts, dressing based on extra virgin olive oil and lemon juice. **Preparation:** Mix all vegetables with quinoa and nuts, season with oil and lemon. **Benefits:** Provides essential nutrients and healthy fats that help maintain a balanced internal environment and promote detoxification.
- *Dinner - Purifying Soup of Vegetables and Legumes.* **Ingredients:** Cauliflower, broccoli, zucchini, carrots, lentils, garlic, onion, homemade vegetable broth, herbs such as rosemary and thyme. **Preparation:** Cook vegetables and lentils in vegetable broth with garlic, onion, and herbs until soft. **Benefits:** A light and nutritious dinner that helps cleanse the body, stimulates liver function, and improves digestion.
- *Snacks - Snacks based on Fresh Fruit and Nuts.* **Ingredients:** Seasonal fruit (apples, pears, citrus fruits) and a handful of walnuts or almonds. **Benefits:** They provide sustained energy and nutrients without weighing down the digestive system, helping to maintain a balanced pH.
- *Drinks during the day - Alkaline Water with Lemon and Ginger.* **Ingredients:** Water, juice of half a lemon, and a few slices of fresh ginger. **Benefits:** It promotes detoxification, stimulates metabolism, and keeps the body hydrated, which is essential for eliminating organs' adequate functioning.

Integrating these strategies and recipes into everyday life makes it possible to create an internal environment conducive to purification, improve digestion, and promote cell regeneration. In this way, you help maintain an internal balance that enhances overall health and increases energy and vitality levels, allowing you to live healthier and more consciously.

Infusions and decoctions to expel excess mucus

Ginger and Lemon Infusion

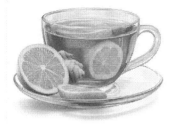

Prep time: 5 min, Cooking time (infusion): 7 min,
Ingredients:

- 3-4 slices of fresh ginger
- Juice of half a lemon
- 250 ml boiling water
  Instructions:
1. Bring the water to a boil.
2. Add the ginger slices to a cup.
3. Pour boiling water over the ginger.
4. Leave to infuse for 7 minutes.
5. Strain the infusion and add the lemon juice.

Chamomile and Mint Infusion

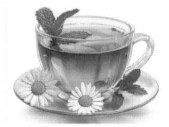

Prep time: 5 min, Cooking time (infusion): 7 min,
Ingredients:

- 1 teaspoon dried chamomile flowers
- 5-6 fresh mint leaves
- 250 ml boiling water
  Instructions:
1. Bring the water to a boil.
2. Place the chamomile flowers and mint leaves in a cup.
3. Pour the boiling water over the ingredients and cover the cup.
4. Leave to infuse for 7 minutes.
5. Strain and drink the hot infusion.

Eucalyptus and Thyme Herbal Tea

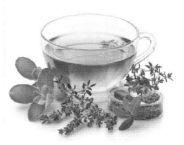

Prep time: 5 min, Cook time (infusion): 8 min,
Ingredients:

- 1 teaspoon dried eucalyptus leaves
- 1 teaspoon dried thyme leaves
- 250 ml boiling water
  Instructions:
1. Bring the water to a boil.
2. Combine the eucalyptus and thyme leaves in a cup.
3. Pour boiling water over the ingredients.
4. Cover and leave to infuse for 8 minutes.
5. Strain and consume the hot brew to rid your lungs of excess mucus.

Nettle Herbal Tea

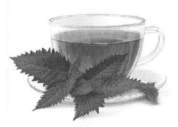

Prep time: 5 min, Cooking time (infusion): 10 min,
Ingredients:

- 1 teaspoon dried nettle leaves
- 250 ml boiling water
  Instructions:
1. Bring the water to a boil.
2. Place the nettle leaves in a cup.
3. Pour boiling water over the leaves and cover the cup.
4. Leave to infuse for 10 minutes, then filter.

Green Tea and Ginger Infusion

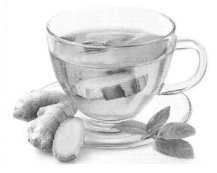

Prep time: 5 min, Cooking time (infusion): 7 min,
Ingredients:

- 1 green tea bag (or 1 teaspoon loose green tea leaves)
- 2-3 slices of fresh ginger
- 250 ml boiling water
  Instructions:
1. Bring the water to a boil.
2. Place the green tea bag and ginger slices in a cup.
3. Pour boiling water over the ingredients and leave to infuse for 7 minutes.
4. Remove the sachet and strain the slices, then drink the hot infusion.

Mallow decoction

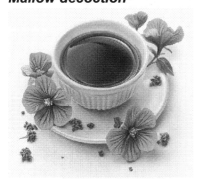

Prep Time: 5 min, Cook Time: 10 min,
Ingredients:

- 1 teaspoon dried mallow flowers
- 250 ml boiling water
  Instructions:
1. Put the mallow flowers in a saucepan with 250 ml of water.
2. Bring to a boil and let it simmer for 10 minutes. Filter and drink hot.

Sage and Rosemary Herbal Tea

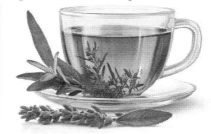

Prep time: 5 min, Cook time (infusion): 8 min,
Ingredients:

- 1 teaspoon dried sage leaves
- 1 teaspoon dried rosemary leaves
- 250 ml boiling water
  Instructions:
1. Bring the water to a boil.
2. Put the sage and rosemary leaves in a cup.
3. Pour boiling water over the herbs and cover the cup.
4. Leave to infuse for 8 minutes, then filter and drink the hot infusion.

Lemon Balm and Ginger Herbal Tea

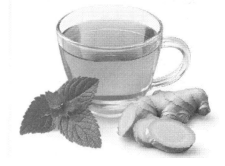

Preparation time: 5 min, Cooking time (infusion): 7 min,
Ingredients:

- 1 teaspoon dried lemon balm leaves
- 2-3 slices of fresh ginger
- 250 ml boiling water
  Instructions:
1. Bring the water to a boil.
2. Place the lemon balm leaves and ginger slices in a cup.
3. Pour boiling water over the ingredients and leave to infuse for 7 minutes.
4. Strain the infusion and drink hot.

These recipes for herbal teas and decoctions are designed to help expel excess mucus, both from the lungs and the digestive tract. By integrating these infusions into your daily routine, you can stimulate diuresis, improve circulation and contribute to the purification of the body, thus creating a cleaner internal environment that is conducive to cell regeneration. Each recipe offers specific properties to relieve mucus buildup, reduce inflammation, and support the body's natural defenses.

Strategies to strengthen the immune system without drugs

Strengthening the immune system naturally means adopting a holistic approach that promotes the entire body's health without resorting to chemical drugs in the first instance. This choice is based on the belief that a body nourished by wholesome foods, supported by herbal remedies and a balanced lifestyle, can prevent many diseases and respond better to infections. The goal is to combat pathogens and create an unfavorable internal environment for viruses and bacteria, keeping the body's pH in an optimal range and reducing inflammation.

A strong immune system is the key to preventing acute and chronic diseases and ensuring a better quality of life. When the body has adequate immune defenses, it can quickly recognize and neutralize external agents, such as viruses, bacteria, and toxins. Conversely, a weakened immune system can pave the way for recurrent infections and persistent inflammation, which can lead to degenerative or autoimmune diseases in the long term. Conventional drugs, while often necessary in acute or critical situations, can have side effects, interfere with hormonal and metabolic balance, and, in some cases, do not act on the root causes of the malaise. Furthermore, the excessive use of drugs can lead to resistance phenomena and a progressive weakening of the immune response. In this context, reducing the intake of chemical drugs, when not strictly essential, means promoting a more sustainable approach for the body based on prevention and the natural strengthening of defenses. Natural remedies are based on the synergistic action of phytochemical compounds present in plants, capable of modulating the immune system and supporting health in an integrated way. The absence of synthetic chemicals reduces the risks of unwanted side effects and, at the same time, offers nutritional and anti-inflammatory support that helps maintain a balanced internal environment. This approach, based on prevention and the promotion of healthy habits, aims to strengthen the body, acting on the causes of many diseases rather than simply suppressing their symptoms.

Dr. Sebi argued that most diseases derive from an internal imbalance, often due to excess acidity and mucus, and that a natural and purifying approach represents the most effective way to prevent and combat numerous diseases. According to his philosophy, using medicinal herbs, alkaline foods, and detoxification practices allows you to restore a favorable body pH, reduce inflammation, and provide the immune system with the necessary support to carry out its task. Dr. Sebi also highlighted the importance of reducing the use of chemical drugs, which can alter hormonal balance and weaken the body's natural defenses in the long term.

Choosing natural remedies and a predominantly plant-based diet also positively impact the environment. A diet rich in fruits, vegetables, and whole grains reduces resource consumption and greenhouse gas emissions compared to a diet rich in industrial and animal-based products. In addition, using medicinal plants from sustainable cultivation and the reduced use of synthetic drugs help preserve ecosystems and biodiversity, promoting a model of well-being that respects the planet.

To strengthen the immune system in a simple, effective, and fast way, it is helpful to adopt an alkaline diet based on whole foods, fruits, vegetables, and legumes, maintain a balanced internal pH, and provide the body with essential nutrients. Integrating medicinal herbs such as Echinacea, Astragalus, or Reishi into your daily routine can stimulate natural defenses and reduce inflammation, especially if accompanied by constant hydration with quality water, preferably alkaline, perhaps enriched with lemon or ginger, to promote purification. Intermittent fasting and detox periods are also helpful in giving "rest" to the digestive system and activating autophagia mechanisms, limiting the accumulation of toxins. On the stress management front, yoga and meditation help keep cortisol levels under control, while moderate physical activity – even walks or stretching sessions – stimulates circulation and improves tissue oxygenation. Finally, reducing exposure to harmful substances by limiting processed foods and harsh household chemicals helps create a healthier body environment and sustainably supports the immune system.

Supporting scientific studies

Several scientific studies conducted in recent years have focused on the effects of a more alkaline diet and lifestyle, showing how a reduction in acid load can positively influence various aspects of health. The following research, published in trade journals and based on different population samples, shows that a diet rich in fruits, vegetables, and whole grains – often associated with a lower intake of animal proteins and processed foods – helps regulate the body's acid-base balance, reduce inflammation and support metabolic functions. Although everyone has unique characteristics and further confirmation may be needed, these studies offer a fascinating insight into the preventive and therapeutic potential of the individual.

Remer T, Manz F (Journal of Environmental and Public Health, 2012) – In this review, the authors analyzed the impact of a diet rich in alkalizing foods on metabolic parameters and kidney function, highlighting that a diet with a low acid load can promote the balance of internal pH, helping to reduce risk factors for some chronic diseases.

Adeva-Andany MM, Fernández-Fernández C, Mouriño-Bayolo D, et al. (European Journal of Nutrition, 2016) – This study investigated the relationship between dietary acidity and the onset of metabolic disorders, showing that an excessive intake of acidifying foods (processed meats, refined sugars) can negatively affect inflammatory and oxidative processes, while a more alkaline diet is protective.

Zhu H, Cao L, Xu C, et al. (Nutrients, 2018) – Research that examined how increased consumption of alkalizing fruits and vegetables can improve endothelial function and reduce oxidative stress in individuals at risk of cardiovascular disease. The results indicate a significant correlation between the intake of alkalizing minerals (such as potassium and magnesium) and cardiovascular health parameters.

Doyle L, Wood R (Frontiers in Public Health, 2020) – Observational study on a group of adults with prediabetes who, after adopting an alkaline lifestyle (based on vegetables, fruits, legumes, and whole grains), showed an improvement in the glycemic profile and a reduction in systemic inflammation. The authors emphasize the importance of supplementing nutrition with adequate hydration and moderate physical activity.

Wyss M, Kistler B, Stadelmann M (PLoS One, 2019) – In this investigation of patients with chronic kidney disease, researchers found that a diet low in acidifying foods and rich in plant foods helped slow the progression of kidney damage and maintain better control of urinary pH, with positive effects on blood pressure as well.

CHAPTER 16: NATURAL REMEDIES FOR THE MOST COMMON INFECTIONS

Infections, whether viral, bacterial or fungal in origin, are a recurring challenge for everyone's health. Often, symptoms, such as fever, sore throat, cold, and inflammation, interfere with daily activities and, if neglected, can lead to more serious complications. Fortunately, nature offers a wide range of remedies, including medicinal herbs, detox protocols, and healthy habits that can support the immune system and promote healing. In this chapter, we will explore simple and safe approaches to dealing with the most common infections, with an emphasis on how to treat colds, flu, bacterial and fungal infections, tonsillitis, and recurrent sore throats, as well as presenting natural protocols for rapid recovery from acute infections.

The proposed approach is based on three fundamental principles: prevent, support and purify. Prevention means adopting daily habits that strengthen the immune system, such as a nutrient-dense diet, adequate hydration and stress management techniques. Supporting means resorting to herbs and medicinal plants that have antiviral, antibacterial and antifungal properties, without forgetting the importance of adequate rest. Finally, purifying consists of the use of detox protocols and detoxification practices that help the body get rid of toxins and metabolic waste, accelerating the healing process. With these integrated strategies, the need for synthetic drugs can be reduced and longer-lasting well-being can be promoted.

How to Treat Colds and Flu Naturally

Colds and flu are common viral infections that particularly affect the respiratory system. When the body is already under stress or weakened, these viruses find a favorable ground to proliferate. A natural approach to counteracting them involves acting on several fronts: boosting the immune system, reducing inflammation and supporting the body in the healing phase. Echinacea, for example, is known for its immune-boosting compounds that help speed up the body's response against viruses. Similarly, infusions of ginger and lemon, rich in antioxidants and substances that promote mucus thinning, can relieve respiratory symptoms and help keep the body in an alkaline state. It is also essential to follow a light diet rich in liquids, such as vegetable broths, purifying herbal teas and fresh fruit, which does not weigh down the digestive system. Adequate rest, then, allows the body to focus its energy on fighting the infection, accelerating healing and reducing the risk of complications.

Vitamins and minerals play a crucial role in strengthening the immune system, especially during times of infectious stress such as colds and flu. Vitamin C, for example, is a powerful antioxidant that protects cells from oxidative stress and stimulates the production of white blood cells, which are essential for fighting viruses. Vitamin D, on the other hand, regulates the immune response and promotes the function of macrophages, cells that are critical for the elimination of pathogens. Minerals such as zinc and selenium are equally important: zinc supports numerous enzymatic and immune processes, contributing to hormone synthesis and cell repair, while selenium aids in the conversion of inactive thyroid hormone into active thyroid hormone and protects cells from oxidative damage. Together, these micronutrients work synergistically to boost the body's natural defenses, making it better able to prevent and fight infection. Purifying broths and soups are an excellent solution to support hydration and thin mucus, facilitating its elimination from the respiratory tract and digestive system. These warm and light meals, prepared with fresh, whole ingredients, not only provide essential nutrients, but also help to warm the body and stimulate circulation. For example, a vegetable broth made from carrots, celery, onion and ginger not only provides vitamins and minerals, but thanks to ginger, with its anti-inflammatory properties, it also promotes better digestion and a reduction in mucus. Similarly, a mixed vegetable soup with an addition of legumes offers a rich source of fiber and vegetable protein that supports the immune system, helping to keep the body purified and well hydrated. These dishes are especially good during the early stages of a cold or flu, as they help soothe an irritated throat and provide the body with the energy it needs to fight off the infection.

Immune-stimulating herbs, such as Echinacea and Astragalus, have long been used to reduce the duration and severity of flu symptoms and to strengthen immunity. Echinacea is particularly known for its ability to stimulate the production of white blood cells and activate immune cells, contributing to a faster response against viruses. It can be taken in the form of herbal teas, tinctures or supplements, and is ideal at the beginning of a flu episode to help the body contain the infection. Astragalus, rich in immunomodulating polysaccharides, helps to reinvigorate the immune system, especially in times of stress and fatigue, and promotes better resistance to respiratory infections. This herb, typical of traditional Chinese medicine, can be consumed in decoctions or supplements and has been shown to be effective in reducing the duration of symptoms and promoting faster recovery. Incorporating these immune-boosting herbs into your daily routine, along with a cleansing diet and stress management techniques, is a natural and comprehensive approach to supporting your body during flu season and keeping your immune system in a state of optimal alertness.

Natural strategies against bacterial and fungal infections

Infections of bacterial or fungal origin often result from an imbalance of the microbiota and an acidic internal environment rich in metabolic waste. To prevent and fight these infections naturally, it is essential to create an environment that is unfavorable for the proliferation of pathogenic bacteria and fungi. A purifying and alkaline diet, rich in fiber and antioxidants, helps maintain the pH balance and support the processes of elimination of toxins. Herbs such as garlic, thyme, and oregano have antibacterial and antifungal properties due to their essential oils and polyphenols, which hinder the growth of unwanted microorganisms. At the same time, the use of probiotics and prebiotics supports beneficial gut flora, making it more difficult for pathogens to take root and improving immune function. Finally, managing stress and ensuring adequate rest are key elements in preserving a reactive immune system and preventing the recurrence of infections.

Home Remedies for Tonsillitis and Sore Throat

Recurrent tonsillitis and sore throat can be caused by viruses, bacteria, or a combination of both. In any case, inflammation of the tonsils and oropharyngeal mucosa leads to pain, difficulty swallowing and often a feverish state. A very effective home remedy consists of gargling with warm water and sea salt, which help disinfect the area and reduce swelling. Equally useful are sage and lemon infusions, known for their antiseptic and soothing properties: sage helps reduce inflammation, while lemon offers a boost of vitamin C. Applying warm compresses to the neck can relieve the sensation of pain, while anti-inflammatory herbal teas based on chamomile, ginger or rosemary help reduce irritation. At a preventive level, it is important to avoid foods and drinks that are too cold or rich in refined sugars, which can aggravate inflammation, and to maintain constant hydration to support the body's natural defenses.

Honey and propolis

Honey and propolis, products of the hive, are known for their extraordinary antibacterial and soothing properties. Honey is rich in enzymes, antioxidants, and natural antibacterial substances that can help reduce inflammation and inhibit the growth of harmful bacteria. When applied to the sore throat, honey forms a protective film that calms pain, reduces itching and stimulates the healing process of damaged mucous membranes. Propolis, on the other hand, contains bioactive compounds such as flavonoids and phenolic acids, which offer a powerful antibacterial, antiviral, and anti-inflammatory effect. These compounds help protect the respiratory tract, preventing infections from worsening and facilitating healing. Together, honey and propolis create a very effective natural remedy to relieve sore throats, reduce irritation and strengthen local immune defenses, representing a valid alternative to traditional pharmacological treatments.

Hot drinks with lemon and ginger

Hot drinks made from lemon and ginger are particularly popular for their dual beneficial effect: warming and anti-inflammatory. Lemon, despite being acidic in concentrated form, has an alkalizing effect once metabolized, helping to rebalance the body's internal pH. In addition, lemon is a rich source of vitamin C, which is crucial for immune support and protecting cells from oxidative damage. Ginger, on the other hand, contains gingerols and shogaols, compounds known for their anti-inflammatory properties and ability to stimulate circulation. When combined in a hot beverage, these ingredients work synergistically to soothe irritated mucosa, thin mucus, and aid in respiratory detoxification. Not only does this blend relieve sore throats, but it also helps to reduce congestion, improve digestion, and provide a warming effect that helps calm the body during times of cold or flu. These beverages are a simple, natural and highly effective remedy to improve comfort during respiratory infections, promoting a cleaner and less inflamed indoor environment.

Herbs and medicinal plants to fight fever and inflammation

Fever is a physiological response of the body that helps fight pathogens, raising the core temperature to slow viral or bacterial replication. However, a fever that is too high or prolonged can cause discomfort and complications. Some medicinal herbs offer valuable support in controlling fever and inflammation. Turmeric, with its curcumin, is a powerful anti-inflammatory and antioxidant that can help modulate the immune response. Elderberry, rich in anthocyanins, acts especially in the case of viral infections and supports the immune system. Licorice root has emollient and anti-inflammatory properties, useful for soothing irritated mucous membranes. Supplementing these plants in the form of herbal teas, decoctions or liquid extracts, perhaps together with a light and fluid-rich diet, promotes tissue recovery and regeneration, without necessarily resorting to synthetic drugs.

1. Ginger and Turmeric Herbal Tea

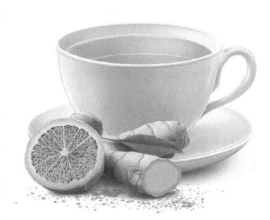

Preparation time: 5 min, Infusion time: 10 min,
Ingredients:

- 3-4 slices of fresh ginger
- 1/2 teaspoon turmeric powder (or a small piece of fresh turmeric)
- 250 ml boiling water
- A pinch of black pepper (to increase curcumin absorption)
- Honey (optional, for sweetening)

Instructions:

1. Bring 250 ml of water to a boil.
2. Put the ginger slices and turmeric in a cup.
3. Pour boiling water over the ingredients and add a pinch of black pepper.
4. Cover the cup and let it steep for 10 minutes.
5. Strain the infusion and, if desired, add a teaspoon of honey.

Gingerols in ginger and curcumin in turmeric possess powerful anti-inflammatory and antioxidant properties, helping to regulate body temperature and reduce inflammation.

2. Elderberry and Linden Infusion

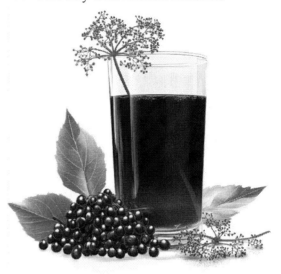

Preparation time: 5 min, Infusion time: 10 min,
Ingredients:

- 1 teaspoon dried elderflower
- 1 teaspoon dried lime blossoms
- 300 ml boiling water
- A slice of lemon (optional)

Instructions:

1. Bring 300 ml of water to a boil.
2. Place the elderflower and linden tree in a teapot or cup.
3. Pour the boiling water over the ingredients, cover and leave to infuse for 10 minutes.
4. Strain the brew and, if desired, add a slice of lemon for a refreshing touch. Elderberry and linden have diaphoretic properties that promote sweating, helping to lower fever and rid the body of toxins accumulated during infections.

3. Green Tea and Rosemary Infusion

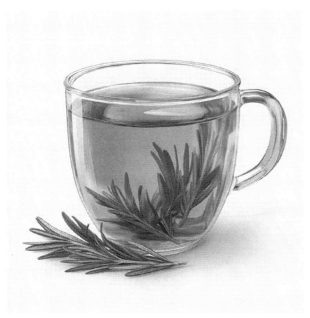

Preparation time: 5 min, Infusion time: 7 min,

Ingredients:

- 1 green tea bag (or 1 teaspoon loose green tea leaves)
- 1 teaspoon dried rosemary leaves
- 250 ml boiling water

  Instructions:
1. Bring 250 ml of water to a boil.
2. Place the green tea and rosemary in a cup.
3. Pour boiling water over the ingredients and let it steep for 7 minutes.
4. Remove the sachet or strain the leaves, then drink the hot infusion.

Green tea is rich in catechins, a type of polyphenol, while rosemary contains antioxidant compounds such as rosmarinic acid.

4. Cold Compress with Anti-Inflammatory Herbal Tea

Preparation time: 10 min, Application time: 15 min,

Ingredients:

- 1 cup of an anti-inflammatory herbal tea (you can use the Ginger and Turmeric Herbal Tea prepared previously)
- A clean cloth or gauze
- A plastic bag (to keep the infusion on the cloth)

Guidelines:

1. Prepare a cup of Ginger and Turmeric Herbal Tea as per the previous recipe and let it cool to room temperature.
2. Dip the clean cloth or cheesecloth into the infusion, squeezing out the excess liquid slightly.
3. Apply the compress to the affected area (for example, on the chest to make breathing easier or on the neck to relieve a sore throat) and leave it on for 15 minutes.
4. Repeat 2-3 times a day, as needed, for continuous relief. The local application of the infusion helps reduce inflammation and calm irritated mucous membranes, facilitating the expulsion of mucus and improving respiratory function through direct contact with the active ingredients.

5. Citrus and Kiwi Smoothie

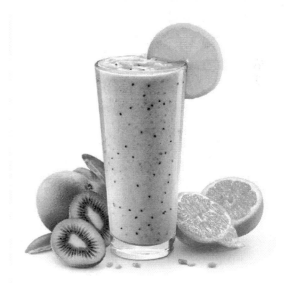

Prep Time: 7 min,

Ingredients:

- 1 peeled orange
- 1 kiwi, peeled
- 1/2 lemon squeezed
- 1 tablespoon of honey (optional)

- 200 ml of cold water or coconut water
- Ice (optional)

Instructions:
1. Put all the ingredients in the blender.
2. Blend until smooth and homogeneous.
3. Serve immediately, adding a few ice cubes if desired. Citrus fruits and kiwi are rich in vitamin C, which strengthens the immune system and helps reduce oxidative stress. This smoothie promotes purification, contributes to a balanced internal pH and supports cell regeneration, facilitating the elimination of excess mucus.

6. Mallow and Chamomile decoction

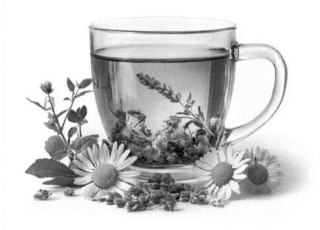

Prep Time: 5 min, Cook Time: 10 min,
Ingredients:

- 1 teaspoon dried mallow flowers
- 1 teaspoon dried chamomile flowers
- 250 ml of water

Instructions:
1. Put the mallow and chamomile flowers in a saucepan with 250 ml of water.
2. Bring the water to a boil and let it simmer for 10 minutes.
3. Strain the decoction and drink hot or at room temperature.

Mallow is known for its soothing and emollient properties, while chamomile has a calming and anti-inflammatory effect. This decoction helps to thin the mucus in the respiratory tract and digestive tract, relieving irritation and contributing to an overall cleansing action.

7. Licorice and Ginger Infusion

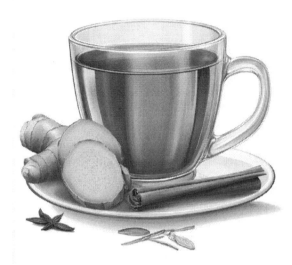

Preparation time: 5 min, Infusion time: 8 min,
Ingredients:

- 1 tsp dried licorice root
- 2-3 slices of fresh ginger
- 250 ml boiling water

Instructions:
1. Bring the water to a boil.
2. Put the licorice root and ginger in a cup.
3. Pour boiling water over the ingredients and leave to infuse for 8 minutes.
4. Strain and drink the hot infusion. Licorice has emollient and soothing properties that help reduce irritation of the mucous membrane, while ginger stimulates circulation and offers an anti-inflammatory action. Together, these ingredients support detoxification and promote the expulsion of excess mucus.

8. Thyme and Oregano Herbal Tea

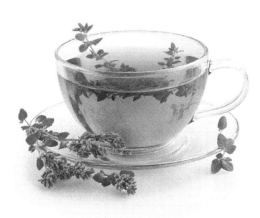

Preparation time: 5 min, Infusion time: 7 min,
Ingredients:

- 1 teaspoon dried thyme leaves
- 1 teaspoon dried oregano leaves
- 250 ml boiling water

Instructions:
1. Bring the water to a boil.
2. Place the thyme and oregano in a cup.
3. Pour boiling water over the herbs and let it steep for 7 minutes.
4. Strain and drink the hot infusion.

Benefits:
Thyme and oregano are rich in essential oils with antimicrobial and anti-inflammatory properties. This infusion stimulates diuresis, promotes purification and helps eliminate excess mucus, improving respiratory function.

9. Peppermint and Eucalyptus Herbal Tea

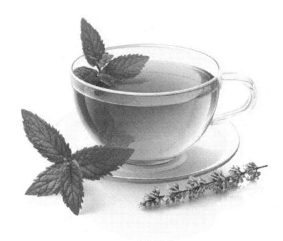

Preparation time: 5 min, Infusion time: 8 min,
Ingredients:

- 1 teaspoon dried peppermint leaves
- 1 teaspoon dried eucalyptus leaves
- 250 ml boiling water

Instructions:
1. Bring the water to a boil.
2. Place the peppermint and eucalyptus leaves in a cup.
3. Pour the boiling water over the ingredients and cover the cup.
4. Leave to infuse for 8 minutes, then filter and drink. Peppermint has a cooling and anti-inflammatory effect, while eucalyptus is known for its expectorant and decongestant properties. Together, they help clear the airways of excess mucus and make breathing easier.

10. Sage and Lemon Infusion

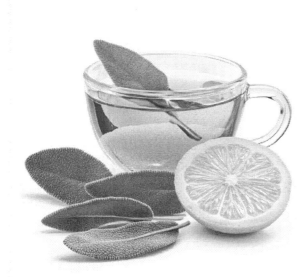

Preparation time: 5 min, Infusion time: 7 min,
Ingredients:

- 1 teaspoon dried sage leaves
- Juice of half a lemon
- 250 ml boiling water

Instructions:
1. Bring the water to a boil.
2. Place the sage leaves in a cup.
3. Pour boiling water over the leaves and let it steep for 7 minutes.
4. Strain the infusion, add the lemon juice and drink hot. Sage is known for its anti-inflammatory and antibacterial properties, while lemon helps maintain an alkaline environment and promotes purification. This infusion is ideal for reducing congestion and facilitating mucus expulsion, improving breathing and supporting the immune system.

11. Chamomile and Lavender Herbal Tea

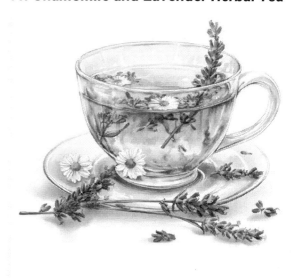

Preparation time: 5 min, Infusion time: 7 min,
Ingredients:

- 1 teaspoon dried chamomile flowers
- 3-4 drops of lavender essential oil (make sure to use only edible oil or diluted properly)
- 250 ml boiling water

Instructions:
1. Bring the water to a boil.
2. Put the chamomile flowers in a cup and add the lavender drops.
3. Pour in the boiling water, cover and let it steep for 7 minutes.
4. Strain the infusion and drink slowly.

Benefits:
Chamomile has a calming and soothing effect, while lavender, thanks to its anti-inflammatory and relaxing properties, helps reduce stress and promotes cleansing of the respiratory tract. This infusion, therefore, supports the purification of mucus and improves respiratory function.

12. Ginkgo Biloba and Ginger Herbal Tea

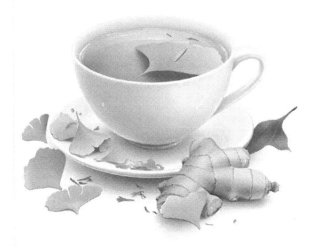

Preparation time: 5 min, Infusion time: 8 min,
Ingredients:

- 1 teaspoon dried ginkgo biloba leaves
- 2-3 slices of fresh ginger
- 250 ml boiling water

Instructions:
1. Bring the water to a boil.
2. Place the ginkgo biloba leaves and ginger slices in a cup.
3. Pour in the boiling water and let it steep for 8 minutes.
4. Strain the infusion and drink hot. Ginkgo biloba is known to improve circulation and protect cells from oxidative damage thanks to its antioxidants, while ginger stimulates digestion and anti-inflammatory action. This infusion helps to promote the flow of mucus, facilitating the elimination of toxins and improving breathing.

Detox protocols to recover quickly from acute infections

When the body faces an acute infection, the production of toxins and metabolic waste greatly increases, straining the elimination organs such as the liver, kidneys, and intestines. A well-structured detox protocol, which includes practices such as intermittent fasting, purifying herbal teas and abundant hydration, can facilitate the process of disposing of these harmful substances. In particular, the intake of draining herbs (dandelion, birch, nettle) and the use of light vegetable broths help to support diuresis and remove waste products more quickly. This integrated approach reduces the toxic load that the body must manage, speeding up recovery and preventing the recurrence of infections. Combined with adequate rest and stress control, the detox protocol allows you to restore internal balance and strengthen the immune system, promoting a shorter convalescence and a better quality of life.

Targeted intermittent fasting is a strategic approach that allows the body to undertake short periods of abstinence from food, during which autophagy mechanisms are activated, a natural process by which cells eliminate damaged components and accumulated toxins. This period of food "rest" promotes cell regeneration and helps the body recover more quickly after an infection. At the same time, the intake of purifying herbal teas such as dandelion, birch and nettle specifically supports the liver and kidneys, essential organs for the elimination of toxins. These plants stimulate diuresis and promote liver function, facilitating the purification process and helping to create a less inflamed internal environment.

A further enhancement of the detox process can be achieved through dry brushing and the use of the sauna. Dry brushing, carried out with a natural bristle brush, stimulates lymphatic circulation, promoting the drainage of liquids and the elimination of toxic residues from the skin. The sauna, on the other hand, induces deep sweating, which helps to expel toxins and improve blood circulation, further strengthening the body's natural defenses.

A liquid and light diet, which involves the consumption of vegetable broths and centrifuges, provides essential nutrients in a gentle way, facilitating the recovery of the digestive system and accelerating recovery after an infection. These "soft" foods reduce the digestive load, allowing the system to focus on cell regeneration and restoring metabolic balance.

Finally, effective post-illness stress management, through practices such as meditation and relaxation techniques, is crucial for reducing cortisol levels. A reduced level of this stress hormone not only promotes tissue repair but also helps to restore hormonal balance and support an optimal immune response.

The integrated approach proposed by Dr. Sebi, which combines intermittent fasting, purifying herbal teas, dry brushing, liquid nutrition and stress management techniques, proves to be extremely functional and successful. This method works on multiple fronts to eliminate toxins, reduce inflammation, and stimulate cell regeneration, thus creating a clean and well-balanced indoor environment. In doing so, the body not only quickly regains its optimal function after an infection, but also strengthens its immune defenses, preventing future relapses and promoting long-lasting health. Dr. Sebi's philosophy, which emphasizes the importance of an alkaline and purifying environment, therefore proves to be a valuable ally for those who want to adopt a natural and sustainable approach to health.

CHAPTER 17: ANTIVIRAL TONICS AND PURIFICATION PROTOCOLS

We live in an era in which pollution, stress and an unbalanced diet cause our body to accumulate toxins, lowering the immune system. This is why it is important to take care of yourself with a natural approach that helps cleanse and strengthen the body. In this chapter, we will discuss how to prepare antiviral tonics and purification protocols that use alkaline ingredients and natural remedies. These tools can help create an internal environment that is less conducive to the reproduction of viruses and bacteria and more suitable for cell regeneration.

One of the key points is to choose foods and herbs rich in active ingredients such as polyphenols, flavonoids, essential oils and minerals. These ingredients help keep the body's pH balanced, reduce inflammation, and stimulate the natural cell repair process, creating an effective barrier against pathogens.

Along with these ingredients, it is important to follow a complete purification protocol: periods of controlled fasting, purifying herbal teas and a light diet rich in whole foods can help the body get rid of accumulated toxins, promoting the proper functioning of the liver, kidneys, intestines and skin. This method, combined with the intake of alkaline foods, enhances the effectiveness of the treatment, stimulating cell regeneration and improving overall health.

Throughout the chapter, we will see practical recipes for infusions and decoctions, how to use essential oils and prepare natural compresses, and we will learn how to create a simple and natural daily routine to prevent infections. The goal is to offer practical and accessible tools to strengthen the immune system, purify the body and support the metabolism, following the natural and purifying principles that inspire Dr. Sebi's philosophy.

How to make a powerful antiviral toner

An antiviral tonic based on alkaline ingredients is a natural and effective solution to support the immune system and create an internal environment that is less conducive to the proliferation of viruses and bacteria. Knowing this recipe is important because it provides a simple and accessible means of counteracting seasonal infections and, at the same time, helps reduce inflammation and maintain a balanced body pH. Consistent use of an alkaline tonic helps to boost the body's resistance to pathogens, offering daily support that can prove invaluable in times of stress or increased exposure to viruses and bacteria.

The ingredients and main actions of the antiviral tonic:

- **Ginger:** Rich in gingerols, compounds known for their anti-inflammatory and antioxidant properties, ginger helps thin mucus, stimulates circulation, and supports digestion, creating an internal environment that is less conducive to the growth of pathogens.
- **Lemon:** Despite its acidic taste, lemon exerts an alkalizing effect on the body once metabolized. The high vitamin C content promotes the synthesis of antibodies and protects cells from oxidative stress, strengthening the immune system.
- **Turmeric:** Curcumin, the most relevant active ingredient in turmeric, is prized for its powerful anti-inflammatory and antioxidant power. It helps reduce inflammatory processes that can weaken the body and promotes tissue regeneration.
- **Garlic:** Known for centuries for its antibacterial and antiviral properties, garlic contains allicin, a compound that hinders the growth of pathogens. Its regular consumption helps to keep the immune system on alert and support respiratory function.

These ingredients act in synergy, offering several beneficial actions: **strengthening the immune system**, thanks to vitamins and phytochemical compounds that stimulate the production of white blood cells; **reduction of inflammation**, as turmeric and ginger counteract inflammatory processes and protect cells from free radicals; **maintenance of a balanced pH**, favoring an alkaline internal environment that makes it more difficult for viruses and bacteria to settle; **support for digestion and circulation**, which in turn allows for a more efficient distribution of nutrients and defensive substances in the body.

Preparing this antiviral tonic is simple: just combine fresh ginger and garlic (grated or crushed), a teaspoon of turmeric powder (or a piece of fresh root) and the juice of a lemon in warm water, possibly sweetening with a pinch of honey. Taking it consistently, in the morning or when you need it, helps to defend yourself naturally against colds, flu and other infections, while promoting better vitality and lasting well-being.

Specific herbal teas and infusions to stimulate natural defenses

Herbal teas and infusions based on medicinal plants are a simple and pleasant way to support the immune system in a natural way. In addition to providing active ingredients such as immunomodulating polyphenols, flavonoids and polysaccharides, these drinks help maintain a balanced and slightly alkaline internal environment, hindering the proliferation of viruses and bacteria. Sipping immune-stimulating herbal teas regularly, especially during the cold months or during periods of increased stress, not only helps prevent infections such as colds and flu but also offers a moment of relaxation that promotes the reduction of cortisol levels (the stress hormone) and the improvement of general well-being.

Below, a list of the main herbal teas recommended to stimulate the immune system, with instructions on how to prepare them:

Echinacea herbal tea

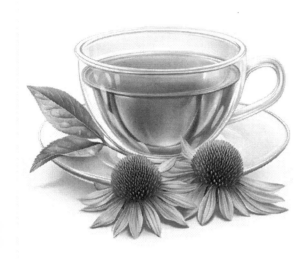

Elderflower and berries, rich in anthocyanins and antioxidants, strengthen the immune system and can reduce the duration of flu symptoms. For preparation, combine a teaspoon of dried flowers with 250 ml of boiling water, leave to infuse for about seven to eight minutes, then strain. For a more incisive effect, combine elderflower with peppermint or thyme leaves, resulting in a mix that is particularly effective against colds and congestion.

Astragalus Herbal Tea

Echinacea increases the production of white blood cells and activates immune cells, allowing the body to react more quickly to external threats. To prepare the herbal tea, use a teaspoon of dried root or leaves in 250 ml of boiling water. Pour the Echinacea into a cup, cover and let it steep for ten minutes, then strain and drink hot. Taking two to three cups a day during periods of increased exposure to viruses, such as in the winter months or during times of fatigue, can intensify immune support.

Elderberry infusion

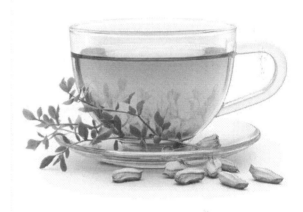

Astragalus is known for its high content of immunomodulatory polysaccharides, which can stimulate the immune response and improve resistance to respiratory infections. It is prepared using a teaspoon of dried root in 250 ml of water, placed in a saucepan starting from cold water. Bring to a boil and simmer for 10-15 minutes, then strain. Consuming one or two cups a day for two to three weeks gradually strengthens defenses, especially in times of stress or seasonal changes.

Rosehip Herbal Tea

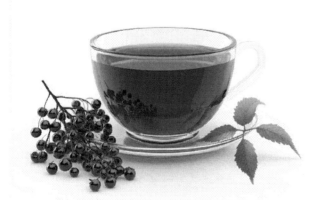

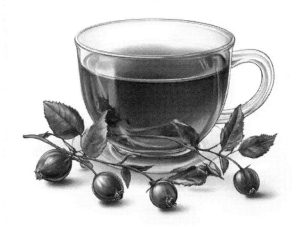

Nettle and dandelion support the liver and kidneys in eliminating toxins, creating a cleaner internal environment that is favorable to the immune response. To make this herbal tea, combine a teaspoon of dried nettle leaves and one teaspoon of dried dandelion root in 300 ml of boiling water, leave to infuse for ten minutes and filter. One cup a day offers a constant purifying action, useful for supporting natural defenses.

Thyme and Rosemary Herbal Tea

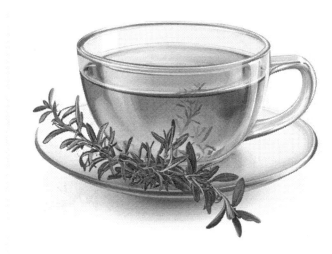

Rosehip, thanks to its high vitamin C content, is an excellent ally for the immune system and to counteract oxidative stress. Put a teaspoon of dried berries in 250 ml of boiling water, cover and leave to infuse for about ten minutes, then filter. To enhance the antioxidant effect, you can add a slice of lemon or a pinch of grated fresh ginger.

Nettle and Dandelion Herbal Tea

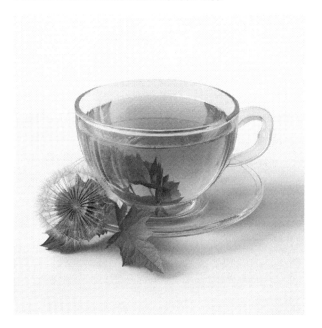

Thyme and rosemary contain essential oils and antioxidants with antimicrobial properties, which protect cells from oxidative stress and contribute to a reactive immune system. Combine a teaspoon of dried thyme and one teaspoon of dried rosemary in 250 ml of boiling water, cover and leave to infuse for about eight minutes, then filter. If you want a balsamic effect, add a few drops of eucalyptus essential oil (food-grade) or a slice of fresh ginger, to amplify the soothing properties and clear the respiratory tract.

Regularly take immune-stimulating herbal teas and infusions

Consuming these drinks consistently helps to provide the body with natural active ingredients that strengthen the immune system, limit inflammation and support the balance of internal pH. Integrating herbal teas into your daily routine, especially during periods of greatest risk (winter or prolonged stressful situations), reduces the likelihood of contracting infections and accelerates healing in the event of seasonal ailments. In addition, the ritual of preparing and enjoying herbal tea itself helps to reduce stress, promoting mental relaxation which in turn boosts the immune system.

Purification programs to rid the body of viruses and toxins

A well-structured purification program is an effective way to help the body rid itself of toxins and waste that, over time, can weaken the immune system and promote the proliferation of viruses. The aim is to stimulate the body's natural self-healing capacity, providing the liver, kidneys, intestines and skin with the necessary support to eliminate harmful substances and restore a clean and balanced internal environment. Through the integration of practices such as short fasts, light and nutritious foods, purifying herbal teas and moderate physical activity, it is possible to reduce oxidative stress, improve lymphatic circulation and stimulate autophagy processes, which allow cells to remove damaged components.

Below, an example of a 60-day purification program, divided into weekly phases, is presented to guide you in the process of eliminating toxins and strengthening the immune system. Remember that this program is only a guideline and should be tailored to your personal needs, lifestyle, and health condition. Before embarking on a detox journey, it is advisable to consult a qualified professional.

60 Day Purification Program

Week	Main Objective	Key activities	Notes
1-2	Start and Preparation	- Adopt a light and purifying diet: prefer fruit, vegetables, whole grains and legumes.	Gradually reduce processed foods and acidifiers.
		- Increase hydration: drink at least 2 liters of water a day, preferably alkaline water with lemon or ginger.	
		- Start with short periods of intermittent fasting (e.g., 12 hours of overnight fasting).	
3-4	Detox Activation	- Increase intermittent fasting periods (up to 14-16 hours of overnight fasting).	Introduce gradually.
		- Consume purifying herbal teas: dandelion, milk thistle, birch and nettle, 1-2 cups a day.	Alternate herbal teas to vary the benefits.
		- Start dry brushing activities to stimulate lymphatic circulation, at least 3-4 times a week.	

5-6	Enhancing the elimination of toxins	- Integrate alkaline foods: fruits, vegetables, legumes, nuts and seeds into every meal, to maintain a balanced internal pH.	
		- Practice daily light physical activity, such as walking or yoga, to support circulation and the elimination of toxins.	
		- Use sauna or weekly steam baths to increase sweating and rid the body of toxic residues.	
7-8	Strengthening of the Immune System	- Continue with the purifying diet and increase the intake of herbal teas and infusions.	
		- Introduce the use of decoctions of draining herbs, e.g. decoction of licorice or mallow, to further support detox processes.	
		- Focus on rest: Make sure you get at least 7-8 hours of sleep per night and practice relaxation or meditation techniques.	
9-10	Consolidation and Monitoring	- Assess progress and, if necessary, adjust the eating plan to maintain pH balance and support cell regeneration.	
		- Increase the intake of foods rich in fiber and antioxidants to facilitate intestinal purification.	
11-12	Maintenance and Prevention	- Continue with detox practices and maintain hydration and regular physical activity.	Build a daily routine.
		- Integrate a daily routine of cleansing herbal teas, dry brushing and short intermittent fasts to prevent the accumulation of toxins in the long term.	

This 60-day program is designed to help the body rid itself of accumulated toxins and strengthen its natural defenses, creating an internal environment conducive to cell regeneration and infection prevention. By adopting practices such as intermittent fasting, regular intake of cleansing herbal teas, physical activity, and stress management, the body can significantly improve the function of its excretory organs – liver, kidneys, intestines, and skin. It is essential to remember that everybody is unique: adapt this program according to your personal needs, your work commitments and your state of health. With patience and perseverance, you will notice significant improvements in your energy, digestion and resistance to infections, in line with the natural and purifying principles promoted by Dr. Sebi's philosophy.

Essential oils and natural compresses to soothe the symptoms of infections

Essential oils are a valuable ally in quickly relieving the symptoms of infections, thanks to their powerful antimicrobial and anti-inflammatory properties. These oils, derived from aromatic plants, act both directly against viruses and bacteria, and by soothing irritation and congestion of the respiratory tract. Applying them in warm compresses or a room diffuser can help create a relaxing atmosphere, reducing discomfort and speeding up the healing process. In parallel, natural wraps made with herbs or clay offer local relief, improving circulation and promoting the elimination of toxins. These techniques, when integrated into a daily routine, provide complementary support to conventional therapy and help manage symptoms effectively and naturally.

Eucalyptus Essential Oil

Eucalyptus essential oil is particularly loved by those looking for natural remedies to improve breathing and air quality at home. Instead of resorting to chemical sprays or over-the-counter medications, many people find eucalyptus to be a gentle but effective ally. By adding three or four drops to a room diffuser, you can create a balsamic atmosphere that promotes the decongestion of the respiratory tract, reducing the sensation of a stuffy nose. If you prefer a topical application, you can dilute the same amount of essential oil in a carrier oil (such as almond or coconut oil) and gently massage into your chest or back. This method is particularly popular with those who want relaxing support and a soothing effect during periods of colds or allergies. Thanks to its antibacterial and anti-inflammatory properties, eucalyptus helps to maintain a healthier home environment, especially in cold seasons or in the presence of high humidity.

Oregano Essential Oil

Oregano essential oil is known for its strong antimicrobial and antiviral properties, so much so that it is considered a sort of "natural antibiotic". Diluting two or three drops in a carrier oil allows you to create a compress to be applied to the affected areas (such as the throat or chest) for a warming and purifying effect. Those who prefer room diffusion can add the same amount to a diffuser, to benefit from the intense aroma of oregano and purify the air in the home. This solution is particularly appreciated by those looking for natural alternatives to fight colds and respiratory infections without resorting to too many drugs. In addition, oregano is often associated with a feeling of comfort and protection, making it appealing to those who want a more welcoming home environment.

Tea Tree Essential Oil

For those who follow a health- and environmentally conscious lifestyle, tea tree essential oil is a must-have in your "natural pharmacy". By adding two or three drops to a diffuser, you can purify the air and reduce the presence of pathogens, thanks to its antifungal and antibacterial properties. If you prefer topical use, dilute the tea tree in a carrier oil and apply it to the skin to relieve minor irritation or impurities. This remedy is particularly popular with those looking for solutions for acne or to soothe insect bites, as its antimicrobial action works quickly. Many people, especially moms looking for natural alternatives, appreciate tea tree for its versatility and fresh scent, associated with a sense of cleanliness and well-being.

Lavender Essential Oil

Lavender is the essential oil preferred by those who love to recreate a relaxing and enveloping atmosphere at home. By using three or four drops in a diffuser, a delicate scent spreads that helps reduce stress and promotes a night's rest. When diluted in a carrier oil, lavender lends itself to light massages on tight or contracted areas, such as the shoulders and neck, offering a calming effect that many people find helpful after a busy day of work or childcare. In addition, lavender supports the immune response in an indirect way: a more serene and relaxed state of mind makes the body more reactive and less prone to seasonal illnesses or stress-related disorders.

Green Clay Wrap

Green clay is an amazing resource for those looking to eliminate toxins and reduce inflammation in a gentle yet effective way. By mixing the clay powder with water until a homogeneous paste is formed, a compress is created that can be applied to various parts of the body (such as chest or back) for ten to fifteen minutes. During this time, the clay absorbs impurities, stimulates local circulation and gives a feeling of freshness. This treatment is particularly popular with those who want a home "spa" effect, as green clay is known for its remineralizing qualities and ability to rebalance the skin. In addition, people with an active lifestyle appreciate clay for its decongestant action on muscles and joints, especially after exercise.

Purifying Herbs Pack (Chamomile and Rosemary)

Chamomile and rosemary, prepared in a strong herbal tea, offer a combined action of calm and purification. Chamomile soothes irritation, while rosemary stimulates circulation and acts as a tissue tonic. Once cooled, the infusion can be used to soak a clean cloth to be applied to the affected areas for about fifteen minutes. Those with sensitive skin or looking for a gentle remedy against swelling and redness will find in this pack an excellent natural solution. In addition, the pleasantness of the aroma makes the application experience more enjoyable, promoting a moment of relaxation and self-care.

Sage and Mint Wrap

For those who struggle with excess mucus or localized inflammation, a concentrated infusion of sage and mint is an ideal combination. Just one teaspoon of each herb in 250 ml of boiling water, let it steep for about eight minutes. Once cooled, the infusion can be used for a ten-fifteen-minute compress on the desired area. Sage is prized for its anti-inflammatory and astringent properties, while mint offers a refreshing and invigorating effect. Many find relief in using this remedy to decongest the chest or nose, especially during periods of colds or allergies, as the combined action of the two herbs helps to thin the mucus and improve local circulation, promoting a feeling of immediate well-being.

How to Create a Daily Routine to Prevent Infections

Preventing infections means adopting healthy habits daily that work synergistically to strengthen the immune system and keep the body in balance. To create an effective routine, it is essential to start the day with a good glass of alkaline water, perhaps enriched with lemon or ginger, which helps stimulate the detoxification system and maintain a favorable internal pH. Drinking enough throughout the day is essential to promote the elimination of toxins through urine and sweat.

Another key component is nutrition: preferring fresh, whole and organic foods – such as fruits, vegetables, legumes and whole grains – provides the body with essential nutrients and antioxidants that strengthen the immune system and counteract inflammation. Avoiding processed foods, refined sugars and acidifying foods contributes to creating an internal environment that is less conducive to the proliferation of viruses and bacteria.

Dedicating moments to rest and exercise is equally important. Even simple daily activities such as walking, stretching or yoga sessions not only improve circulation and tissue oxygenation, but also help reduce stress levels. Practicing relaxation techniques, such as meditation or deep breathing, allows you to lower cortisol levels, the stress hormone, and promote mental well-being that reflects positively on the immune system. Finally, regularly supplementing herbal teas and alkaline tonics, along with small purification protocols such as controlled intermittent fasting or the consumption of purifying decoctions, helps keep the body in a state of constant cell regeneration and detoxification. These practices support the excretory organs – liver, kidneys, intestines and skin – and help reduce the accumulation of toxins and metabolic waste, making the body more resistant to attacks by viruses and bacteria.

Adopting a daily routine that integrates all these recommendations is crucial to prevent infections naturally and sustainably. With small but constant changes in daily habits, it is possible to create a balanced internal environment, which boosts the immune system and promotes better overall health, protecting the body from external threats and promoting long-term well-being.

CHAPTER 18: NATURAL CARE FOR SKIN AND HAIR

Skin and hair are often considered a "business card" of our state of health: when they appear bright, strong, and well hydrated, they reflect the internal balance of the body and the proper functioning of vital processes such as circulation, cell regeneration, and hormone production. On the contrary, skin problems or weakened hair can indicate an imbalance that involves not only the external surface but also metabolism, diet, and lifestyle. In this chapter, we will explore the natural approach to caring for your skin and hair, drawing on the principles of Dr. Sebi and holistic medicine. We will analyze how a healthy and alkalizing diet, rich in essential nutrients and free of inflammatory substances, can improve the external appearance by acting from the inside. At the same time, we will see how herbal supplements, herbal remedies, and daily practices can enhance the action of a balanced diet, helping to maintain skin elasticity, counteract premature aging, and strengthen hair. In addition to nutritional claims, we will address the importance of restful sleep, stress management, and choosing natural cosmetics free of harsh chemicals. We will discover, for example, how simple vegetable oils or herbal masks can offer a deeply nourishing and regenerating treatment for the skin and hair without exposing us to the potential side effects of conventional products. We'll also talk about how small, everyday gestures – such as dry brushing, scalp massage, or proper weather protection – can prove decisive in achieving lasting results.

The natural approach to skin and hair care, in line with Dr. Sebi's thinking, considers the individual in its entirety: every action we carry out externally, from the choice of products to the beauty routine, is intertwined with the quality of nutrition, emotional balance and the health of internal organs. This integrated vision makes self-care a transformative experience in which improving one's external appearance becomes a way to take care of the body and mind. In the following paragraphs, we will, therefore, delve into strategies and tips to nourish and protect the skin and hair naturally, promoting well-being that radiates from within and is reflected in the brightness and vitality of each individual cell.

How to counteract hair loss with alkaline remedies

Hair loss is often the result of internal imbalances, oxidative stress, inflammation, and nutritional deficiencies. The health of the scalp and the strength of the hair follicles depend not only on genetic and hormonal factors but also on the state of our body. An excessively acidic and intoxicated body tends to show signs of discomfort through the skin, hair, and nails, making them more fragile and prone to falling out. Following an approach based on alkaline remedies helps restore the body's biochemical balance, providing cells with all the essential nutrients to regenerate and function optimally. A slightly alkaline body environment promotes better blood circulation, tissue oxygenation, and healthy hair growth, preventing hair weakening and premature loss. A determining factor in scalp health is the supply of alkalizing minerals such as potassium, magnesium, iron, and silicon, which support cell renewal and keratin production. This main protein makes up the hair shaft. A diet rich in alkaline foods helps neutralize internal acidity and promote the elasticity of tissues, including the scalp.

The most beneficial foods to counteract hair loss are those that provide essential nutrients and support scalp health. Leafy greens, such as spinach, kale, and Swiss chard, are vital for their high chlorophyll content and essential minerals, which help nourish follicles and stimulate hair growth. In addition, cucumbers and celery are prized for their moisturizing and detoxifying properties, helping to maintain internal balance and promoting better circulation in the scalp. Avocado and almonds offer a rich source of beneficial fatty acids and vitamin E, which are essential for nourishing and protecting hair roots, while pumpkin seeds and sunflower seeds, rich in zinc, provide the indispensable mineral for strengthening follicles and stimulating growth. Finally, figs and dates, thanks to their iron and silicon content, are excellent for giving strength to the hair and promoting its healthy development. These foods, integrated into a balanced diet, help create an internal environment conducive to hair growth, improving scalp health and reducing the risk of hair loss.

At the same time, it is essential to eliminate or reduce acidifying foods such as refined sugars, dairy products, white flour, and processed meats, which contribute to scalp inflammation and follicular activity reduction. In addition to diet, several topical and herbal remedies help stimulate microcirculation in the scalp, strengthen hair follicles, and prevent hair weakening. One of the most effective is coconut oil, which is known for its antibacterial, antifungal, and nourishing properties. Applying it directly to the scalp before shampooing helps nourish the follicles, prevent dryness, and protect the hair from breakage. Another highly recommended remedy is massage with essential oils, which improves blood circulation and reduces stress-related hair loss. Oils such as rosemary, lavender, and peppermint can be mixed with a carrier oil (jojoba or castor oil) and gently applied in circular motions to stimulate the hair bulbs.

Supplementing alkalizing herbal teas such as nettle and burdock root helps purify the liver and blood, thus improving the nourishment of the scalp and making the hair healthier and more resistant. Stress management is another aspect that should not be overlooked, as high cortisol levels are directly linked to hair loss. Meditation, yoga, and deep breathing can reduce systemic inflammation and restore a hormonal balance for hair growth.

Hair Health

1. **Case of Hair Loss Due to Nutritional Deficiencies:** A person suffering from progressive thinning might experience a noticeable improvement by introducing a daily alkaline smoothie made from spinach, avocado, pumpkin seeds, and almond milk. After a few weeks, the hair would appear firmer, thanks to the increased intake of B vitamins, iron, and zinc.
2. **Case of Hair Loss Linked to Stress and Acidification of the Body:** An individual with high-stress levels and an unbalanced diet could significantly reduce hair loss by adopting a routine based on purifying herbal teas (nettle and burdock), daily meditation, and applications of rosemary essential oil on the scalp. After a few months, thinning would be reduced, and growth would be more vigorous.

Counteracting hair loss naturally requires a comprehensive approach, combining a mineral-rich alkaline diet, nourishing topical remedies, and stress management. Dr. Sebi's philosophy, based on body purification and deep cellular nutrition, offers an effective solution to restore internal balance and promote healthy and lush hair growth. Adopting these principles in your daily routine not only helps prevent hair loss but improves the quality and strength of your hair over time, restoring vitality and well-being to the entire body.

Natural treatments for eczema and psoriasis

Eczema and **psoriasis** are chronic skin disorders with **inflammation, flaking, itching, and redness**, often linked to genetic, immune, or environmental factors. Although their origin is complex and multifactorial, there are **natural strategies** that can help **reduce symptoms and improve skin health**. There are different forms of eczema and psoriasis, each with specific characteristics. Some people may have **atopic eczema**, which is more common in children and linked to allergic reactions. In contrast, others may have **plaque psoriasis**, which is characterized by scaly, red patches. In some cases, it can be challenging to identify your condition accurately. **Consulting a dermatologist is essential to receive a correct diagnosis and understand the natural approach that best suits your case**.

One of the most critical aspects of the natural treatment of these conditions is **nutrition**, which can **reduce systemic inflammation and support skin regeneration**. Following an **antioxidant and alkaline** diet helps to strengthen the immune system and keep the skin healthy. Eliminating inflammatory foods, such as dairy products, refined sugars, and processed foods, and including fresh foods **rich in minerals and phytonutrients** helps reduce the frequency and intensity of skin manifestations.

In parallel, **topical natural remedies** can offer **immediate relief**, soothe irritation, and promote skin healing. **Aloe vera** is particularly effective due to its **calming and moisturizing** properties. At the same time, **coconut oil** helps to restore the skin barrier and protect the skin from secondary infections. Herbs such as **chamomile and calendula** are used as infusions or ointments to reduce redness and itching. At the same time, **oatmeal compresses** have an emollient and soothing effect, which helps relieve burning and dryness.

In addition to these remedies, it is essential to maintain **a gentle skincare routine**, avoiding harsh soaps and choosing products **that are free of irritating chemicals**, such as parabens and synthetic fragrances. **Constant hydration** with natural plant oils helps protect the skin and reduce water loss, a crucial factor for those suffering from eczema or psoriasis.

1. **Case of Atopic Eczema and Sensitive Skin:** A child or adult with **atopic eczema** might benefit from applying **aloe vera gel** daily and using **jojoba oil** after showering to seal moisture and reduce dryness. A diet **rich in leafy greens, pumpkin seeds, and avocados** provides **alkalizing minerals** that help rebalance the immune response.
2. **Case of Plaque Psoriasis and Intense Flaking:** Those suffering from plaque psoriasis, with dry and scaly areas of skin, may get relief from baths with oatmeal and lavender essential oils. Applying calendula ointment and coconut oil helps reduce itching and irritation. In contrast, a diet free of dairy and refined sugars can help reduce the frequency of flare-ups.
3. **Case of Stress Eczema and Inflamed Skin:** For a person who experiences **eczema due to stress**, in addition to topical remedies, it is helpful to integrate relaxation practices such as **meditation, yoga, and mindful breathing**. Regular intake of **chamomile and nettle herbal teas** helps reduce inflammation and improve the body's response to stress, promoting skin improvement over time.

The natural treatment of **eczema and psoriasis** requires a **holistic approach** that combines **nutrition, topical natural remedies, and stress management**. The alkaline diet and the support of medicinal herbs can play a crucial role in reducing symptoms and improving skin quality. **Consulting with a dermatologist to identify the specific type of eczema or psoriasis and choosing the most suitable treatment is crucial for the best results.** Following a natural protocol and a healthy lifestyle can **restore your skin's balance and promote long-term well-being.**

Herbal Masks & Lotions Recipes

Skin and hair care through herbal masks and lotions is a natural and effective way to nourish, regenerate, and protect tissues. Using 100% natural and chemical-free ingredients allows the skin to be deeply hydrated, reduces inflammation, and promotes cell regeneration, improving the skin's and hair's overall appearance. The active ingredients in herbs and vegetable oils are potent antioxidants, soothing and rebalancing, capable of counteracting skin aging, rebalancing sebum production, and strengthening the hair from the root. Making masks and lotions at home allows you to tailor them to your specific needs, choosing ingredients targeted at your skin and scalp concerns.

For example, a moisturizing and soothing face mask can be made by mixing aloe vera gel, coconut oil, and a few drops of lavender essential oil. This combination is perfect for dry and sensitive skin, thanks to its emollient and calming properties. Another helpful preparation is a toning chamomile and calendula lotion, ideal for irritated and reactive skin, as it helps reduce redness and inflammation. For hair health, a nourishing mask based on castor oil, argan oil, and rosemary infusion is an excellent treatment to stimulate scalp circulation, strengthen hair follicles, and counteract hair loss. Preparing these recipes with fresh and natural ingredients is essential. Mix them carefully and store them in dark glass containers to protect them from light and keep their active ingredients intact.

Integrating these preparations into your daily beauty routine and combining them with a balanced diet and wellness practices can transform the quality of your skin and hair, improving its brightness, elasticity, and strength over time.

5 Herbal Masks and Lotions Recipes

Moisturizing and Soothing Face Mask with Aloe Vera and Lavender

Ingredients:
- 2 tablespoons of aloe vera gel
- 1 tablespoon of organic coconut oil
- 3-4 drops of lavender essential oil

Preparation and use:

1. Mix the ingredients until smooth.
2. Apply the mask to a clean face and leave it on for 15-20 minutes.
3. Rinse with warm water and gently pat the skin dry with a soft towel.

Aloe vera calms and regenerates the skin, coconut oil deeply moisturizes, while lavender has relaxing and anti-inflammatory properties.

Toning Lotion with Chamomile and Calendula

Ingredients:
- 1 cup chamomile tea
- 1 cup of calendula infusion

Preparation and use:

1. Prepare two separate infusions with chamomile and calendula, leaving them to infuse for 10-15 minutes.
2. Filter and mix the two liquids, adding apple cider vinegar if necessary.
3. Transfer the lotion to a spray container and use it morning and night as a facial toner.

Chamomile and calendula have soothing, anti-inflammatory and rebalancing properties, ideal for reddened or reactive skin.

Strengthening Hair Mask with Castor Oil and Rosemary

Ingredients:
- 1 tablespoon castor oil
- 1 tablespoon of argan oil
- 1 cup rosemary infusion
- 5 drops of peppermint essential oil

Preparation and use:

1. Make a rosemary infusion and let it cool.
2. Mix the oils with the infusion and apply the mixture to your scalp.
3. Massage gently and leave on for 30 minutes before washing your hair with a natural shampoo.

Castor oil stimulates hair growth, rosemary strengthens follicles and peppermint improves circulation.

Brightening Mask with Turmeric and Almond Milk

Ingredients:
- 1 teaspoon turmeric powder
- 1 tablespoon of almond milk
- 1 teaspoon of natural honey

Preparation and use:

1. Mix the ingredients until creamy.
2. Apply the mask to your face and leave it on for 10-15 minutes.
3. Rinse with warm water, being careful not to stain your clothes with turmeric.

Turmeric has antioxidant and brightening properties, while almond milk moisturizes and soothes the skin.

Soothing Wrap with Oats and Jojoba Oil

Ingredients:
- 2 tablespoons of oatmeal
- 1 tablespoon jojoba oil
- 2 tablespoons warm water

Preparation and use:

1. Mix the oatmeal with the water until you have a soft paste.
2. Add the jojoba oil and mix well.
3. Apply to the skin and leave on for 15 minutes, then rinse with warm water.

Oats soothe irritated skin and jojoba oil helps restore the natural lipid film.

PART 6: DR. SEBI'S SPECIAL MANUALS

CHAPTER 19: DR. SEBI'S FOOD LIST – APPROVED FOODS

In this chapter, we will explore in detail the official list of foods recommended by Dr. Sebi, a fundamental reference point for those who want to follow an alkaline diet and adopt a healthier and more conscious lifestyle. Dr. Sebi's philosophy of maintaining an alkaline internal environment is based on the belief that many chronic ailments and degenerative diseases result from excess acidity and a buildup of toxins in the body. To counteract this condition, its diet focuses on natural, non-hybrid, and additive-free foods to provide the body with essential nutrients while promoting purification and cell regeneration.

Within this chapter, you will find the so-called Dr. Sebi Food List, a collection of fruits, vegetables, whole grains, legumes, and other foods that, according to his studies and experience, help to keep the body's pH slightly alkaline. These foods, rich in minerals, fiber, and antioxidants, provide the immune system with concrete support, facilitating the elimination of metabolic waste and making the body less susceptible to infections. On the contrary, acidifying or hybrid foods – i.e., the result of unnatural crosses and often poor nutrients – are not recommended because, again, according to Dr. Sebi's vision, they could weigh down the body and slow down self-healing processes.

One of the main objectives of this chapter is to guide you in identifying alkaline foods and avoiding those that, due to their composition or cultivation and processing methods, can compromise the internal balance. You will learn to **read labels** critically, recognizing products that, despite appearances, contain acidifiers, preservatives, and additives. You will find practical advice on how to shop smartly, choose quality ingredients, and verify the origin and genuineness of the products.

This chapter can become a constant point of reference for you. Whenever you have doubts about what to put in the cart or want to check if a food complies with Dr. Sebi's principles, you can consult these pages and find a complete guide. In addition, we will devote space to **concrete strategies** to simplify the preparation of meals without sacrificing taste and variety. You'll find out where to buy fresh, whole foods, even if you don't have a lot of time, and how to organize your pantry so that you always have foods compatible with the alkaline diet on hand.

Finally, we will also discuss the **differences between natural foods and hybrid foods** and why Dr. Sebi suggested avoiding them: hybridized varieties, often created to improve yield or resistance to pests, may be less rich in nutrients and less suitable for a diet oriented towards well-being and body purification. We will, therefore, delve into how to recognize these differences and orient oneself towards foods that are as pure and vital as possible.

Whether you're just starting your journey to an alkaline lifestyle or want to dive deeper into Dr. Sebi's advice, this chapter will give you a comprehensive overview of approved foods, the reasons behind them, and the benefits of introducing them into your daily routine. Get ready to discover a new vision of food, where every choice is a step towards internal balance, vitality, and long-term health.

Dr. Sebi's official list is fruits, vegetables, grains, and legumes

Below are 25 foods generally recognized as compatible with Dr. Sebi's approach, with brief notes on their properties and main phytochemical aspects. The aim is to provide an overview of foods that, according to the philosophy of an alkaline and cleansing diet, can help maintain a balanced internal environment and support immune function.

1. **Amaranth (cereal)** – Rich in high-quality protein, fiber, and minerals such as calcium and iron, it supports red blood cell production and bone health, thanks to polyphenols and squalene that help counteract oxidative stress and promote cell regeneration.
2. **Quinoa (cereal)** provides all the essential amino acids, as well as magnesium and phosphorus, essential for energy and muscle function; the flavonoids present, such as quercetin and kaempferol, offer anti-inflammatory and antioxidant action.
3. **Teff (cereal)** – A high fiber and iron content supports bowel regularity and red blood cell production; its polyphenols help reduce inflammation and regulate metabolism.
4. **Navy beans (legumes)** are a vegetable protein and fiber source that promotes cholesterol control and intestinal regularity. Saponins and phytosterols help support the immune system and lipid metabolism.
5. **Chickpeas (legumes)** offer a good amount of protein, fiber, and complex carbohydrates that release energy gradually; the isoflavones and phenolic compounds present can reduce inflammation and help maintain hormonal balance.
6. **Lentils (legumes)**: Rich in iron, protein, and B vitamins, lentils support energy production and nervous system health; tannins and flavonoids help protect cells from oxidative damage.
7. **Spinach (vegetable)** – Contains folic acid, iron, and calcium, promoting red blood cell formation and bone health, with lutein and zeaxanthin protecting the eyes and fighting inflammation.
8. **Swiss chard (vegetables)** provide vitamin K, magnesium, and potassium, essential for blood clotting and electrolyte balance. At the same time, betalains offer anti-inflammatory and antioxidant properties.
9. **Okra (vegetable)** – Its high soluble fiber content promotes digestion and blood sugar control. At the same time, mucilage and phenolic compounds help maintain a balanced internal pH.
10. **Zucchini (vegetable)** – Low in calories and rich in B vitamins and minerals, they promote hydration and purification, supported by carotenoids and phenolic compounds that act against inflammation.
11. **Blueberries (fruits)** are excellent sources of antioxidants and vitamin C. They protect the heart and blood vessels, and the anthocyanins present counteract inflammation and support brain health.
12. **Figs (fruits)** – Rich in fiber, they promote intestinal regularity and microbiota balance; the flavonoids and organic acids help reduce inflammation and promote an alkaline environment.
13. **Persimmons (fruits)** – They provide vitamins A and C, which are helpful for healthy skin and the immune system, thanks to tannins and carotenoids that act as powerful antioxidants.
14. **Papaya (fruit)** – Known for the presence of papain, an enzyme that facilitates the digestion of proteins and supports intestinal purification; carotenoids and phenolic compounds help promote immune function and cardiovascular health.

15. **Prunes (fruits)** – High fiber content that regulates intestinal transit and stabilizes blood sugar levels; phenolic acids and flavonoids offer antioxidant and anti-inflammatory effects.
16. **Avocado (fruits/vegetables)** – Rich in monounsaturated fats, B vitamins, potassium, and fiber, it supports cardiovascular health and inflammation control; phytosterols and antioxidants promote cell regeneration and cholesterol regulation.
17. **Lime (fruit)** – Contributes vitamin C and minerals to aid digestion and maintain pH balance; limonene and flavonoids help boost liver function and eliminate toxins.
18. **Cherries (fruits)** are a source of vitamins A and C, potassium, and fiber. They support joint health and reduce inflammation, and anthocyanins offer antioxidant properties that protect the cardiovascular system.
19. **Oranges (fruits)** are rich in vitamin C, which is crucial for the immune system and collagen synthesis; flavanones, such as hesperidin and carotenoids, reduce inflammation and improve blood vessel health.
20. **Dates (fruits)** Provide natural sugars, fiber, potassium, and magnesium, which provide energy and support muscle health; phenols and flavonoids help regulate inflammation and protect cells from oxidative damage.
21. **Brazil Nut (seeds)** – One of the best sources of selenium, essential for thyroid function and powerful antioxidant support; phytosterols and phenolic compounds support cardiovascular health and lipid regulation.
22. **Nuts (seeds)** – Rich in omega-3s, proteins, and fibers, they promote the well-being of the heart and brain; polyphenols and tocopherols help reduce inflammation and promote cell repair.
23. **Onion (vegetable)** – Contains quercetin and sulfur compounds that support the immune system and liver function; essential oils and flavonoids help reduce inflammation and have antimicrobial properties.
24. **Bell peppers (vegetables)** are an excellent source of vitamin C, potassium, and beta-carotene, which support eye and immune health; capsaicin in hot peppers and carotenoids offer antioxidant and thermogenic benefits.
25. **Arugula (vegetable)** – Provides B vitamins, vitamin K, and minerals such as iron, contributing to blood circulation and clotting; glucosinolates and flavonoids help regulate inflammation and strengthen the immune system.
26. **Bananas** are a natural source of potassium and fiber, and they help regulate blood pressure and provide sustained energy.
27. **Pears** – Rich in fiber and antioxidants, they support digestion and promote a balanced internal environment.
28. **Pineapple** – Contains bromelain, an enzyme that aids digestion and reduces inflammation.
29. **Guava** – Excellent vitamin C and fiber source, boosts immunity, and supports digestive health.
30. **Watermelon** – Rich in water and antioxidants, it helps to hydrate the body and eliminate toxins.
31. **Melon** – A source of vitamins A and C, it promotes hydration and supports immune function.
32. **Grape** – Rich in resveratrol and anthocyanins, it offers powerful antioxidant properties and supports cardiovascular health.
33. **Almonds** contain healthy fats, vitamin E, and magnesium, which are beneficial for heart health and immune support.
34. **Pecans** are a source of omega-3 and antioxidants; they help reduce inflammation and improve metabolism.
35. **Pumpkin Seeds** – Rich in zinc and magnesium, they support immune function and help maintain strong bones and muscles.
36. **Sunflower Seeds** – Offer vitamin E and selenium, natural antioxidants that protect cells from oxidative stress.

37. **Whole Grain Oats** – Excellent source of soluble fiber, helps regulate blood sugar and stabilizes energy levels.
38. **Wholemeal Spelt** – Rich in protein, fiber, and B vitamins, it promotes digestion and metabolic well-being.
39. **Whole Barley** – Contributes to maintaining a healthy gut due to its high fiber content and essential nutrients.
40. **Brown Rice** – A source of complex carbohydrates and fiber, it supports slow digestion and provides consistent energy.
41. **Millet** – Easily digestible cereal, rich in minerals such as magnesium and phosphorus, promotes cell regeneration.
42. **Spirulina** – This seaweed, rich in proteins, vitamins, and antioxidants, helps strengthen the immune system and cleanse the body.
43. **Chlorella** – Green algae rich in chlorophyll is a natural support for detoxification and strengthening of the immune system.
44. **Seaweed (Nori)** – Rich in iodine and minerals, they help keep pH balanced and support thyroid function.
45. **Carrots** – Source of beta-carotene, which is converted into vitamin A, essential for skin and eye health and offers natural antioxidants.
46. **Cauliflower** – Rich in vitamins C and K, it promotes purification and helps reduce internal inflammation.
47. **Broccoli** – Contains sulforaphane, a compound that stimulates cleansing enzymes and offers potent anti-inflammatory properties.
48. **Asparagus** – Rich in fiber and antioxidants, it supports kidney function and aids in the elimination of toxins.
49. **Kale** – A source of vitamins K, C, and A, it promotes cardiovascular health and provides antioxidants that fight inflammation.
50. **Green beans** – Rich in fiber, vitamins, and minerals, they support digestion and contribute to a balanced immune system.

What to eat and what to avoid

Dr. Sebi, known for his approach focused on maintaining an alkaline internal environment, believed many diseases resulted from excess acidity and a buildup of mucus and toxins. According to his philosophy, a diet composed of natural and non-hybrid foods could promote the body's self-healing, supporting the function of the excretory organs (liver, kidneys, intestines, skin) and stimulating the immune system. The idea behind his method is to nourish the body with foods rich in minerals, vitamins, and phytochemicals, avoiding those that promote inflammation and acidification.

Below is a detailed list of what, according to Dr. Sebi, should be privileged and what should be eliminated or reduced to a minimum to achieve and maintain an optimal internal balance.

What to eat

1. **Fresh, alkaline fruits and vegetables:** These foods, especially leafy greens (spinach, chard, arugula) and low-sugar fruits (apples, pears, berries), provide essential fiber, vitamins, minerals, and antioxidants. They help cleanse, support the gut microbiota, and maintain a balanced internal pH, making the body less susceptible to viruses and bacteria.

2. **Whole grains (quinoa, amaranth, teff, spelt, millet)** offer complex carbohydrates, vegetable proteins, and micronutrients such as iron and magnesium. They release energy gradually, control blood sugar levels, and promote bowel regularity, helping to maintain an alkaline environment.
3. **Legumes (lentils, chickpeas, navy beans, peas):** Rich in protein, fiber, and minerals (iron, zinc, selenium), they provide prolonged energy and promote the growth of beneficial bacteria in the intestine, helping to reduce inflammation and improve the immune response.
4. **Seeds and dried fruits (walnuts, almonds, Brazil nuts, pumpkin seeds):** Source of healthy fats, vitamins (E and B), and minerals (magnesium, selenium, zinc). Monounsaturated and polyunsaturated fats protect the heart and modulate inflammation, while micronutrients strengthen the immune system and support hormonal functions.
5. **Algae and marine plants (spirulina, chlorella, nori):** Rich in minerals such as iodine, iron, calcium, and antioxidants. They promote the chelation of heavy metals and cell regeneration, supporting the body's pH balance.
6. **Herbs and spices (ginger, turmeric, oregano, thyme)** contain essential oils and phenolic compounds with anti-inflammatory, antimicrobial, and antioxidant action. They improve digestion, stimulate circulation, and contribute to a more balanced pH, reducing the proliferation of pathogens.

Must-Avoid Items

1. **Red meat and sausages:** Rich in saturated fats and inflammatory substances, these foods can acidify the body and slow down the process of eliminating toxins, promoting chronic inflammation and weakening the immune system.
2. **Dairy products:** Casein and other components can generate excess mucus and increase internal acidity, hindering proper respiratory and digestive function and creating an ideal environment for pathogens to proliferate.
3. **Hybrid and genetically modified foods:** Often low in nutrients and rich in additives, they alter the body's biochemical balance and make tissue regeneration more difficult, straining the immune system.
4. **Refined sugars and industrial sweets** cause glycemic spikes and promote inflammation, which in turn promotes the growth of pathogenic bacteria and fungi. They also strain the pancreas and immune system, increasing mucus production and susceptibility to infection and metabolic disease.
5. **Refined flours and industrial bakery products:** Free of fiber and micronutrients, they cause fluctuations in blood sugar and increase systemic inflammation. The absence of fiber slows down intestinal transit and promotes the accumulation of waste, weakening the immune defenses.
6. **Refined vegetable oils and trans fats:** Refining processes eliminate nutrients and create oxidized fats responsible for inflammation and cellular stress. It is better to use unrefined oils (such as extra virgin olive oil) that retain phenols and antioxidants that are beneficial for an alkaline internal environment.
7. **Sugary and carbonated drinks:** Rich in simple sugars and chemical additives, they promote body acidification and mucus accumulation, increasing the load of toxins and weakening the immune response.
8. **Excess alcohol** impairs liver function and reduces the absorption of vitamins and minerals. It promotes inflammation and slows down cell repair processes, exposing the body to a greater risk of infection.

9. **Refined table salt:** Excess sodium consumption generates water retention and electrolyte imbalance, contributing to internal acidification. Whole sea salt or pink Himalayan salt are preferable, as they offer useful minerals and limit excess sodium.
10. **Industrial foods are rich in additives.** They often contain preservatives, artificial colors, and flavors, which can irritate the digestive system and weaken the immune system. They interfere with proper metabolism, preventing the appropriate elimination of toxins and compromising overall well-being.

Natural Foods and Hybrid Foods: Why Avoid Them

The distinction between natural and hybrid foods is a central theme in Dr. Sebi's philosophy, which considers nutrition a fundamental tool for keeping the body healthy and preventing chronic diseases. According to this view, an alkaline and purified internal environment is essential to counteract the accumulation of toxins and promote cell regeneration. Natural foods, rich in nutrients, are considered the most valid allies to achieve this balance, while hybrid foods – obtained from crosses and genetic manipulations – can deplete the body of minerals and compromise self-healing processes.

Natural foods play a fundamental role in supporting human health, as they grow wild or are cultivated in accordance with nature's rhythms, free from artificial crossbreeding or genetic modifications intended to enhance yield or resistance to pests. In their purest form, fruits, vegetables, legumes, and whole grains maintain a rich concentration of essential nutrients, including minerals, vitamins, fibers, and phytochemicals such as polyphenols and flavonoids, which possess powerful anti-inflammatory, antioxidant, and immunostimulant properties. These bioactive compounds not only contribute to overall vitality but also help sustain a slightly alkaline body pH, a crucial factor in preventing the overgrowth of harmful viruses and bacteria while facilitating the natural detoxification processes carried out by the liver, kidneys, and other excretory organs. By adopting a diet centered on natural foods, individuals can provide their bodies with a broad spectrum of essential nutrients in balanced proportions, avoiding the detrimental accumulation of pesticide residues, chemical additives, and synthetic preservatives often found in conventionally processed foods. This approach fosters improved digestion, enhanced immune function, and long-term metabolic efficiency, allowing the body to regenerate more effectively and maintain a state of equilibrium.

For Dr. Sebi, the consumption of natural, unaltered foods is not just a recommendation but a necessity for achieving optimal health. His philosophy emphasizes that the human body is designed to function best with foods that retain their original, unmodified structure, in harmony with the principles of nature. Selecting fresh, seasonal fruits and vegetables, unrefined whole grains, and sustainably grown legumes is not only beneficial for personal well-being but also contributes to biodiversity and environmental conservation, reducing reliance on harmful agricultural chemicals. In addition, incorporating medicinal herbs and natural spices into one's diet amplifies the protective effects of a nutrient-dense eating regimen, offering continuous support against systemic imbalances that can lead to chronic inflammation and degenerative diseases.

In contrast, hybrid foods—those derived from genetic manipulation and selective breeding—pose a potential threat to health, according to Dr. Sebi. While these foods are often engineered to increase productivity, resistance to pests, and market appeal, they may suffer from diminished nutritional integrity, making them less compatible with human metabolism. Many hybridized crops lack the full spectrum of minerals and essential phytochemicals found in their wild or naturally occurring counterparts. Additionally, they often contain lower fiber content, which can hinder the body's ability to eliminate toxins and impair the self-healing mechanisms necessary for maintaining robust health. For this reason, Dr. Sebi warns against the widespread consumption of overly engineered foods, as their biochemical composition may contribute to systemic acidification, toxin buildup, and metabolic disruptions, ultimately increasing susceptibility to chronic ailments.

To counteract these risks, Dr. Sebi strongly advocates for the selection of whole, natural foods grown through traditional farming methods, free from artificial crossbreeding or genetic alteration. He urges individuals to opt for produce, grains, and legumes that remain true to their original genetic blueprint, ensuring the body receives the complete range of nutrients required for sustaining an alkaline internal environment. In doing so, the body's natural defense and detoxification systems are optimized, reducing the burden on organs such as the liver and kidneys while enhancing immune resilience. Additionally, Dr. Sebi underscores the importance of eliminating processed foods, refined sugars, and mass-produced industrial products from the diet, as these items introduce synthetic chemicals, excessive acidity, and inflammatory compounds that interfere with cellular function and long-term well-being. By adhering to a diet composed primarily of alkaline, nutrient-rich foods, individuals can restore their body's natural equilibrium, improve energy levels, and promote lasting health from within.

A study published in the *Journal of Agricultural and Food Chemistry* examined the nutritional composition of different varieties of fruits and vegetables and found that hybridized varieties, often developed to increase yield or resistance to pathogens, sometimes have lower levels of antioxidants and phytochemicals than their unmodified counterparts. For example, in some cases, hybridized tomatoes show a reduction in levels of lycopene and other carotenoids, which are essential for cell protection, compared to traditional tomatoes.

Another study, conducted and published in the *Journal of Nutrition*, analyzed the nutritional differences between hybridized and non-hybridized apple varieties. It showed that non-genetically modified apples have a more complete nutritional profile, with higher concentrations of vitamin C, anthocyanins, and other antioxidants, which are fundamental in counteracting oxidative stress and supporting the immune system.

These studies provide concrete evidence that genetic manipulation while offering advantages in terms of productivity and resistance to environmental stresses, can negatively impact plants' essential nutrient content and bioactive compounds. This confirms Dr. Sebi's thesis that a diet based on natural, non-hybridized foods contributes to a better supply of micronutrients and a more complete nutritional profile, thus promoting an optimal internal balance and excellent disease resistance.

Understanding the differences between natural foods and hybrid foods is a crucial step in adopting a healthier lifestyle in harmony with Dr. Sebi's principles. Focusing on foods that preserve their original structure intact and respect the natural rhythms of cultivation helps maintain a balanced internal pH, strengthen the immune system, and promote cell regeneration, protecting the body from the onset of chronic diseases.

How to read labels and recognize alkaline foods

Food labels are a valuable source of information that allows you to know the composition of the food you consume. Knowing how to read these labels is essential to identifying ingredients and additives that could negatively affect your health and to choosing foods that are in line with a cleansing and alkaline lifestyle.

Labels are the "business cards" of a product and contain important data such as the list of ingredients, the nutritional content, the presence of allergens, and, in many cases, information on the production method. These directions help you understand what nutrients you are getting into your body and whether the product contains additives or chemicals that could alter the internal pH.

In the United States, the Food and Drug Administration (FDA) establishes precise rules for food labeling, ensuring transparency and safety. At the same time, the EFSA (European Food Safety Authority) has similar tasks to protect the consumer and ensure that the information provided is accurate and up to date. Both agencies require labels to include precise data on nutritional values, ingredients' origin, and additives' presence, allowing you to compare products and choose the most natural and purifying ones. Food regulations are set by national and international laws that impose strict standards for transparency and product safety. For example, in the United States, the Food Labeling and Education Act (FLEA) and subsequent updates in the United States, while in Europe, EU Regulation 1169/2011 establishes how information on food products must be presented. These regulations ensure that each label provides essential details, allowing you to recognize whether a food has been minimally processed or contains additives that could alter its effect on body pH. When we talk about healthy food, we mean foods that provide essential nutrients, are as natural as possible,e and are not subject to manipulation processes that deplete their nutritional profile. Healthy food, such as fruits, vegetables, legumes, whole grains, and some nuts, is generally alkaline or neutral and helps maintain a balanced internal environment, promoting cell purification and regeneration.

Looking to the future, we can imagine a food landscape increasingly oriented towards sustainability, authenticity, and attention to health, in which consumers demand products that reflect these values. The increase in environmental awareness, together with a greater sensitivity towards the impact that food has on the well-being of the body, is pushing both producers and researchers to develop organic farming methodologies and processing systems that keep the nutritional qualities of food intact. This means selecting varieties of plants rich in micronutrients grown without harmful chemicals and with techniques that respect the natural cycles of the soil and ecosystem. In practice, this translates into "minimally processed" foods, i.e., processed as little as possible after harvesting, to preserve fiber, vitamins, minerals, and phytochemicals essential for health as much as possible. In parallel, the most modern dietary formulations of the future focus on increasing the fiber content and reducing saturated fats and refined sugars. On the one hand, increasing dietary fiber helps promote intestinal regularity and maintain a balanced microbiota while promoting a more gradual release of sugar into the blood. On the other hand, the reduced use of simple sugars and poor-quality fats allows you to limit inflammation and avoid glycemic peaks, contributing to a more stable internal pH and a better immune response.

These "future" foods, often labeled as "natural" or "organic," therefore represent a step forward not only for the health of the individual but also for that of the planet. Growing nutrient-rich plants with environmentally friendly methods means reducing the use of water resources, preserving biodiversity, and limiting the impact of chemical fertilizers and pesticides. In this scenario, the vision of a purifying and alkaline diet, which aims to protect food vitality and support the body with a balanced intake of beneficial substances capable of counteracting inflammatory processes and preventing chronic diseases, is perfectly aligned.

Reading food labels carefully allows you to make informed choices: Look for products with simple ingredients, free of additives, and that meet transparency standards established by agencies such as the FDA and EFSA. opt for natural foods, which Dr. Sebi recommends keeping the body in balance, and get ready to discover the food of the future, oriented towards sustainability and well-being. With this information, you'll easily recognize which products promote an alkaline indoor environment and which could compromise your health.

Shopping at the supermarket

1. Preparation and Planning: **Targeted shopping list:** Before leaving home, make a list of the foods you really need, favoring seasonal fruits and vegetables, whole grains, and legumes. This will help you focus on essential purchases and avoid unnecessary or unhealthy products. **Study of local offers and markets:** Find out about supermarket offers or, if possible, visit local markets and shops specializing in organic or regional products. These places often offer fresh, unprocessed foods, ideal for a natural and purifying diet.
2. Selection of Fresh Foods: **Pay attention to seasonality.** Seasonal fruits and vegetables are richer in nutrients and usually grown with lower amounts of pesticides. In addition, their taste and texture are better than those of out-of-season products. **Observation and touch:** Evaluate the appearance of food. The peel of fruits and vegetables should be intact, without bruises or excessive stains. A light touch can help you check for freshness (for example, a zucchini or cucumber should not be too mushy).
3. Label Reading: **Ingredients and Additives:** Ensure the ingredient list is short and free of chemical additives, colorings, or preservatives. Avoid products with acronyms such as E-xxx, which could indicate the addition of potentially irritating or harmful substances. **Provenance and certifications:** Choose organic food or food with quality certifications (such as the European organic label), which guarantee high standards and sustainable production methods.
4. Purchase of Cereals and Legumes: **Prefer wholemeal versions:** Rice, pasta, spelt, barley, and other cereals should be chosen in the wholemeal variant, as they preserve bran and germ and are rich in fiber, minerals, and vitamins. **Integrity and expiration check:** Make sure that the package does not show signs of moisture or breakage and check the expiration date to ensure a fresh product is free of mold or parasites.
5. Choose Quality Vegetable Proteins: **Legumes and oilseeds:** Lentils, chickpeas, beans, peas, pumpkin, sunflower, or chia seeds provide essential protein and micronutrients. Opt for organic versions and, when possible, verify the origin to support transparent and quality supply chains. **Potential purchase of selected animal proteins:** If your diet includes them, prefer lean cuts, extensive or organic farms, and reduce the frequency of consumption to minimize the accumulation of toxins and maintain a balanced body pH.
6. Beware of Fats and Sugars: **Unrefined Oils:** Favor extra virgin olive oil or other cold-pressed oils (such as flaxseed) to ensure healthy fats and beneficial phenolic compounds. **Natural sugars:** Reduce added sugars as much as possible and, when necessary, replace them with natural sweeteners such as honey or maple syrup in small amounts.
7. Storage and Organization: **Food Distribution:** Once at home, organize fresh foods to consume the most perishable foods first. Freeze whole grains and legumes if you can't use them quickly to preserve their nutritional properties. **Cooking and preparation:** Prepare vegetable broths, vegetable or legume-based sauces, and portions of cooked cereals in advance. This way, you'll always have ready-made ingredients for balanced and healthy meals, even when time is short.

These strategies, combined with careful label reading and a deeper knowledge of food production and origin methods, will allow you to shop more consciously. By choosing quality, fresh, and nutrient-rich ingredients, you can more easily follow an alkaline and natural diet, supporting your body in purifying, regenerating cells, and maintaining an internal balance favorable to health.

CHAPTER 20: DR. SEBI STD CURE – NATURAL CURE FOR SEXUALLY TRANSMITTED DISEASES

Sexually transmitted diseases (STDs) are a widespread health problem, often surrounded by fear, stigma and embarrassment. However, knowing and adopting natural healing methods can open new perspectives for preventing and treating these infections, promoting a holistic approach that supports the harmony of the entire body. In this chapter, we will explore Dr. Sebi's approach, which is based on the idea that proper nutrition and targeted internal cleansing of the body are essential for strengthening the immune system and creating an environment less hospitable to pathogens.

Knowing the natural cures for STDs is crucial for several reasons. Firstly, a natural approach can help prevent infections by reducing inflammation and improving immune function through a nutrient-dense diet and alkalising foods. Secondly, the use of herbal and herbal remedies is often less invasive than conventional drug treatments, which can cause unwanted side effects. In addition, many people respond positively to care methods that integrate harmoniously with their lifestyle, offering sustainable solutions that can be easily integrated into their daily routine. A crucial aspect of this approach concerns the knowledge of the main phytochemicals that can benefit healing processes. Among these, flavonoids are known for their antioxidant and anti-inflammatory properties, capable of protecting cells from oxidative damage and modulating the immune response. Terpenes, with their antiviral and antibacterial power, help to create an internal environment that is less conducive to the development of pathogens. In addition, polyphenols, thanks to their purifying action, support the removal of accumulated toxins. At the same time, the alkaloids in some plants help regulate the body's pH, promoting an alkaline environment that, according to Dr. Sebi, is incompatible with the proliferation of diseases. This chapter, therefore, aims to provide a complete and in-depth picture of natural strategies to address and prevent STDs, highlighting how the integration of conscious eating, the support of medicinal herbs, and the targeted use of phytochemicals can contribute to a more balanced and lasting sexual health. The goal is to offer the reader practical tools and in-depth knowledge to make him an active protagonist of his own well-being, in harmony with the laws of nature.

The link between diet and sexually transmitted diseases

A balanced diet nourishes the body and plays a vital role in maintaining hormonal balance and preventing numerous diseases, including sexually transmitted diseases. It is essential to understand how our food affects our immune system, body pH, and, ultimately, our ability to resist infections and hormonal imbalances that can promote the onset of diseases.

Dr. Sebi, known for his philosophy based on the alkaline diet and the use of natural remedies, claimed that the human body if fed with genuine and natural foods, can maintain an ideal internal environment for self-healing. According to him, the presence of excess mucus and an excessively acidic pH represent the perfect conditions for the onset of various diseases, including some types of sexually transmitted infections. In this context, a diet rich in fruits, vegetables, and whole grains – foods that contribute to an alkaline and toxin-free environment – becomes a fundamental weapon for strengthening the immune system and preventing imbalances that can promote infection.

Adherence to set mealtimes is crucial for hormonal balance. In addition to food choice, eating at regular intervals helps regulate the release of hormones, reducing metabolic stress and keeping your metabolism stable. This regular rhythm promotes better digestion, helps avoid blood sugar spikes, and maintains constant energy levels, which is essential for proper immune function and sexual health. In fact, hormonal imbalances can weaken the body's natural defenses, making the body more susceptible to infections, including sexually transmitted ones.

On the other hand, certain foods can contribute to the onset of sexually transmitted diseases indirectly, promoting chronic inflammation and alterations in the balance of internal pH. Processed foods, rich in refined sugars, saturated fats, and chemical additives, increase the acid load in the body, inducing an environment conducive to the proliferation of pathogens. These foods, in fact, not only weigh down the digestive system but can also compromise the body's ability to cleanse itself of toxins and maintain a reactive immune system. On the contrary, a diet based on whole and natural foods promotes a less inflammatory environment. It is more in tune with the body's natural defense mechanisms. Phytochemicals that play a key role in this process include flavonoids, terpenes, and polyphenols. Flavonoids, for example, possess potent antioxidant and anti-inflammatory properties that help protect cells from oxidative stress and modulate immune responses. Terpenes, on the other hand, offer antiviral and antibacterial effects, creating an indoor environment that is less hospitable to pathogens. Finally, polyphenols act as natural purifiers, facilitating the elimination of toxins accumulated in the body and promoting a balanced pH, essential for general health and infection prevention.

Flavonoids

These compounds are known for their powerful antioxidant and anti-inflammatory properties. They protect cells from oxidative stress, counteracting damage caused by free radicals. Thanks to these properties, flavonoids help to modulate the immune system, promoting a balanced response against chronic infections and inflammation. In other words, an adequate intake of flavonoids helps maintain a health-friendly indoor environment, preventing many conditions that can compromise overall well-being.

Terpenes

Terpenes are a large family of aromatic compounds found in essential oils and resins. They possess antiviral, antibacterial, and even anti-inflammatory properties. Terpenes help create an internal environment that is less hospitable to pathogens, supporting the body's natural defenses. Therefore, their presence in many foods and natural preparations contributes to protection against infections and promotes an optimal physiological balance.

Polyphenols

Polyphenols act as natural purifiers, helping the body eliminate accumulated toxins and maintain pH balance. They support cellular functions and, thanks to their anti-inflammatory properties, help prevent the onset of pathological processes related to chronic inflammation. Their synergistic action with flavonoids and terpenes makes polyphenols particularly effective in protecting and regenerating the body.

Interestingly, despite not knowing these scientific terms, Dr. Sebi sensed these substances' importance. He promoted using natural and whole foods – fruits, vegetables, herbs, and grains – which we know today are rich in flavonoids, terpenes, and polyphenols. His approach was based on the idea that nourishing the body with wholesome foods could create an alkaline internal environment rich in vital energy in which the immune system could act efficiently and naturally. Even without in-depth technical knowledge, Dr. Sebi recognized the importance of the active ingredients present in many natural foods, which are essential for preventing diseases and supporting self-healing processes.

Flavonoids, terpenes, and polyphenols are essential compounds that work synergistically to protect cells, reduce inflammation, and support the body's regenerative capacity. Dr. Sebi's approach to a natural, alkalizing diet sensed the presence and importance of these beneficial substances, even though modern terms were not part of his vocabulary. Adopting a diet rich in these compounds ultimately means providing our body with the necessary tools to stay healthy and balanced, promoting healing that starts from within and is reflected in all physical and mental well-being.

Antiviral and antibacterial herbs for the treatment of infections

Antiviral and antibacterial herbs are key pillars in the fight against infections, especially sexually transmitted diseases. These medicinal plants contain active ingredients that effectively counteract viruses and bacteria, reducing the infectious load and supporting the immune system in eliminating pathogens. Taking them frequently, especially in the presence of sexually transmitted infections, can help not only contain and reduce symptoms but also prevent the spread of the disease within the body.

In addition to the main active ingredients, medicinal herbs are rich in a broad spectrum of phytochemicals – such as flavonoids, terpenes, and polyphenols – that act synergistically to provide a double benefit: on the one hand, they act directly against pathogenic microorganisms on the other, they offer secondary benefits in different organs of the body. For example, these antioxidant and anti-inflammatory compounds can help improve circulation, protect cells from oxidative stress, and support the body's overall well-being. In this way, antiviral and antibacterial herbs not only help fight sexual infections but also promote an overall balance, promoting the restoration of health in various body systems. Taking these herbs regularly, preferably in natural preparations such as infusions, decoctions, or tinctures, therefore becomes an effective strategy for preventing and treating infections, holistically supporting self-healing.

Grass	Main Phytochemical	Main disease/condition treated
Burdock	Arctiin and lignans	Viral and bacterial infections; Blood purification
Sarsaparilla	Saponins	Skin and inflammatory infections, immune system support
Cascara Sagrada	Anthocyanones and anthraquinones	Intestinal infections and detoxification support
Nettle	Quercetin (flavonoids)	Urinary tract infections and inflammation
Fucus Vesiculosus	Fucoxanthin	Hormonal imbalances and immune system support (related infections)
Dandelion	Taraxasterol	Liver and digestive problems, with antibacterial effect
Ginger root	Gingerol	Gastrointestinal infections, nausea and inflammation
Licorice root	Glycyrrhizin	Viral infections (e.g. herpes) and anti-inflammatory properties
Lavender	Linalool	Skin infections, inflammation and stress reduction support
Red clover	Isoflavones	Hormonal imbalance-related infections, support during menopause
Aloe Vera	Acemannan and anthraquinone compounds	Skin infections and promotion of scarring
Turmeric	Curcumin	Inflammatory infections, arthritis and immune function support
Echinacea	Chocolate acid	Respiratory tract infections and immune stimulation
Tea Tree (Melaleuca)	Terpinen-4-ol	Skin infections, candidiasis and other bacterial/viral infections
Ginseng	Ginsenosides	Chronic fatigue, immune support and general well-being
Peppermint	Menthol	Respiratory infections and digestive disorders
Rosemary	Carnosol and rosmarinic acid	Nervous system infections and improved circulation
Sage	Rosmarinic acid	Respiratory infections, inflammation and digestive support
Chamomile	Apigenin	Gastrointestinal infections and calming/anti-inflammatory activity
Garlic	Allicin	Cardiovascular infections, natural antibiotics and immune support

Not only do these herbs contain specific active ingredients that act against viruses and bacteria, but they are also rich in numerous other phytochemicals that offer secondary benefits to various organs and systems in the body. Regularly adopting these herbs in natural preparations – such as infusions, tinctures or decoctions – can be a valuable support for the treatment and prevention of infections, including sexually transmitted disorders, thus integrating a holistic approach to health.

Specific detox plans to combat infections

The detox plan proposed here offers a general approach to helping the body get rid of accumulated toxins and strengthening the immune system during a viral infection, promoting self-healing. It is important to remember that this guideline should be tailored to your individual needs, health conditions, and professional opinion. Each organism responds differently, so adopting this path must be gradual and careful.

First, adequate hydration plays a fundamental role: drinking at least 2-3 liters of water a day, perhaps enriched with fresh lemon, stimulates the emunctory system and promotes the elimination of toxins. Water, in fact, acts as a means of transport that allows the body to be purified and cellular functions to be supported during recovery. A plant-based diet is essential to provide the body with vitamins, minerals, and antioxidants. Consuming plenty of fruits, fresh vegetables, whole grains, and legumes helps boost your immune system and maintain a less acidified internal environment by reducing or phasing out processed foods and refined sugars that can disrupt the metabolic balance.

The use of purifying herbs is of central importance in this detox plan. Infusions and decoctions based on plants such as dandelion, milk thistle, and ginger support liver function, improve digestion, and stimulate detoxification, protecting the body from the harmful effects of pathogens. These herbs work synergistically to promote the elimination of toxins, contributing to a cleaner indoor environment and a better ability to defend against infections. In addition to the nutritional aspects, adopting a holistic approach that includes regular meals and mindful eating practices is essential. Setting fixed mealtimes, enjoying food mindfully, and chewing slowly allow optimal digestion and promote the assimilation of nutrients. At the same time, a well-maintained hormonal balance supports the entire purification process. Even moderate physical activity, such as walking, yoga, or stretching sessions, helps improve circulation and promote detoxification through sweat without overly straining the system during recovery.

Immune system support is essential during the detox process. Taking natural supplements rich in vitamins C, D, and zinc can boost the body's defenses, as can the use of green tea or echinacea infusions, which have been shown to reduce the duration and severity of symptoms. Adequate rest and effective stress management through meditation or deep breathing techniques complete this approach, which is crucial for cell regeneration and optimal recovery.

By adopting this detox plan, which acts on several fronts, the elimination of toxins is promoted, the nutrients necessary to support the immune system are provided, and an internal environment is created that is less favorable to the proliferation of viruses and bacteria. Always remember that every organism is unique and that factors such as age, pre-existing medical conditions, lifestyle, and degree of infection require a personalized plan fit. For best results, it is advisable to consult a health professional who can guide the detox path safely and effectively.

Customize your detox plan.

Personalizing a detox plan means recognizing that each body is unique, with different needs related to metabolism, immune status, hormonal imbalances, and food sensitivities. For this reason, starting by evaluating one's biological constitution is essential: those more prone to acidic or inflammatory states can benefit more from more significant supplementation of alkalizing foods and herbs, such as dandelion or milk thistle. At the same time, those who need immune support can favor herbs such as echinacea or sarsaparilla. A step-by-step approach is essential: start with small doses of new foods or infusions, keep a diary to monitor the body's response, and adjust doses accordingly. Integrating this path with specialized advice, proper stress management, and moderate physical activity allows you to create a personalized and sustainable detox plan over time, supporting purification and improving overall well-being.

Effectiveness of purifying herbs in counteracting viral infections

Numerous scientific studies have highlighted the potential of purifying herbs to strengthen the immune system and counter viral infections. Research published in phytotherapy journals has shown that herbs such as dandelion and milk thistle improve liver function and facilitate blood purification, reducing the toxic load that can promote the proliferation of viruses and bacteria. Other studies have confirmed that echinacea stimulates the production of white blood cells, which are essential for a rapid response to infections. In addition, numerous studies have pointed out that polyphenols, present in many herbs, have antioxidant and anti-inflammatory properties, inhibiting viral replication and protecting cells from oxidative stress. This scientific evidence supports the use of purifying herbs as a therapeutic support and an effective preventive tool against viral infections, which aligns with the holistic approach of a natural diet and a healthy lifestyle.

How to get rid of excess mucus

Excess mucus is a key factor in the spread of infections, as it creates an ideal environment for the accumulation of toxins and the proliferation of pathogens, such as viruses and bacteria. According to Dr. Sebi, mucus is not just a symptom but a real barrier that, if not eliminated, hinders the proper functioning of the immune system and promotes the onset of diseases. Let's delve into how to act on this aspect to strengthen the immune system and promote healing.

Mucus is a viscous, gel-like substance produced by the mucous membranes that line numerous internal organs, including the respiratory tract, digestive system, and urogenital system. Under normal conditions, mucus performs fundamental protective functions: it acts as a barrier against pathogens and irritants, lubricates and protects delicate surfaces, and contributes to removing foreign particles through mucociliary clearance. When mucus production is regulated and balanced, the mucosal system operates efficiently to ensure the health of internal organs. However, in the presence of infections, chronic inflammation, or dietary and environmental imbalances, the body can produce excessive mucus. This excess becomes a toxic "manure," trapping bacteria, viruses, and other impurities, preventing the immune system from effectively eliminating them.

The accumulation of mucus is associated with an imbalance in the internal pH: an environment that is too acidic promotes the proliferation of pathogens and reduces the efficiency of natural self-healing mechanisms. When mucus becomes excessive, a barrier hinders the proper circulation of nutrients, restricting their access to cells and compromising vital tissue repair and regeneration processes. At the same time, the body's ability to eliminate toxins through excretory systems (such as the liver, kidneys, and lymphatic system) is impaired, further accumulating harmful substances that fuel inflammation.

This environment of stagnation and toxicity, caused by excess mucus, weakens the immune response and makes the body more vulnerable to infection. Excess mucus becomes a breeding ground for bacteria and viruses, promoting their proliferation and contributing to the persistence or aggravation of infections. In addition, mucus buildup can alter the function of cell receptors and interfere with normal signaling processes between immune system cells, slowing down the body's ability to recognize and react promptly to pathogens. Therefore, keeping mucus production under control is essential to preserve a balanced internal environment and allow the immune system to function optimally. Interventions such as an alkaline diet, constant hydration, and cleansing herbs are helpful strategies to reduce excess mucus and facilitate detoxification, thus helping to strengthen the body's natural defenses and prevent the onset or worsening of infections.

Natural Strategies to Eliminate Excess Mucus

Maintaining adequate hydration is essential to eliminate excess mucus. Drinking plenty of water during the day, perhaps enriched with lemon, and purifying herbal teas based on a dandelion, ginger, or mint helps to thin the mucus, making it more easily eliminated through urine, sweat, and breathing. Warm water with lemon promotes a more alkaline internal environment, counteracting the formation of toxic mucus and stimulating the emunctory system.

Eating a diet rich in fruits, vegetables, and whole grains and avoiding processed foods, refined sugars, and animal products is essential for keeping the body's pH slightly alkaline. According to Dr. Sebi's philosophy, an alkaline internal environment reduces excess mucus formation. It promotes natural self-healing mechanisms, making the body more resistant to inflammation and infection. Medicinal herbs are essential in fighting excess mucus due to their mucolytic, anti-inflammatory, and antibacterial properties. Plants such as nettle and ginger root can help thin mucus and reduce inflammation, while garlic and licorice strengthen the immune system in the fight against infections with their antibacterial and antiviral actions. These remedies directly intervene in the reduction of mucus and provide a series of beneficial phytochemicals for various organs, contributing to overall well-being. Regular physical activity is a key element in facilitating mucus clearance. Light exercises such as a daily walk, yoga sessions, or stretching stimulate circulation and deep breathing, expulsing accumulated mucus and freeing the airways from congestion. The constant movement also supports lymphatic drainage, helping the body eliminate toxins and keep energy levels high.

Mucolytic herbs

Incorporating mucolytic herbs into your daily diet can be a valuable support for respiratory health, helping to naturally thin mucus and clear the airways. A practical approach is to vary their use in different preparations not to weigh down the system but to constantly stimulate it. For example, you can start the day with a dandelion or nettle-based herbal tea, which, besides having mucolytic properties, also supports the body's general purification process. These infusions, consumed regularly, promote better hydration and help maintain an alkaline internal environment, essential for counteracting excess mucus.

Another strategy is to use powdered herbs, such as those made from ginger root or burdock, which can easily be added to smoothies, soups, or salads. In this way, these plants' mucolytic and anti-inflammatory properties are integrated directly into meals without requiring complex preparations. Herbs' versatility also allows you to experiment with combinations that enhance their effect. For example, adding a hint of turmeric to a green smoothie improves the flavor, helps reduce inflammation, and supports detoxification.

In addition, to obtain continuous support for respiratory health, it is advisable to alternate mucolytic herbs during the week to vary the intake of active ingredients and prevent any intolerances. For example, you can use dandelion herbal teas on some days and switch to nettle-based ones on others, supplementing occasionally with herbs such as ginger and licorice, known for their stimulating and soothing properties. This rotation approach allows the respiratory system to be constantly supported, promoting effective purification and helping prevent respiratory problems naturally and sustainably.

Strengthening the Immune System

Clearing excess mucus is only part of the path to well-being—strengthening your immune system to prevent new infections is just as essential. A body free of toxic mucus, adequately hydrated, and fed alkalizing foods functions optimally and repels pathogens. Natural supplements (such as vitamin C, zinc, and probiotics) and regular relaxation techniques (meditation, yoga, mindful breathing) can further enhance the body's natural defenses.

Eliminating excess mucus is essential to create an internal environment conducive to healing and prevent infection onset. Combining constant hydration, an alkaline diet, herbs, and breathing techniques makes it possible to rid the body of accumulated toxins and strengthen the immune system. Despite having no knowledge of modern scientific terms, Dr. Sebi's thoughts intuited that nourishing the body with natural foods and supporting it with herbal remedies was the key to activating self-healing processes. This concept remains a valuable guide for those who want to live harmoniously with nature. Everyone, however, must adapt these strategies to their specific state of health and personal needs, working in synergy with their body to achieve lasting well-being.

CHAPTER 21: DR. SEBI DETOX CLEANSE SMOOTHIES – SMOOTHIES FOR DEEP CLEANSING

Detox smoothies are an extremely practical and versatile tool for those who want to integrate the principles of Dr. Sebi's philosophy in a simple and tasty way. According to his approach, the elimination of toxins is one of the fundamental pillars of maintaining an alkaline and healthy body, and smoothies—rich in fruits, vegetables, and superfoods—become precious allies to promote this deep purification process.

In this chapter, we will find out why smoothies play a central role in the detox routine, which ingredients to select to obtain highly alkalizing and nutritious drinks, and how to combine them to support the liver, intestine, and blood in eliminating waste. We will also delve into the most effective recipes for boosting energy levels, reducing inflammation, and generally promoting daily well-being. The goal is to provide the reader with practical and easy-to-adopt solutions so that the purifying action can occur gradually but constantly, accompanying the body towards an increasingly balanced state of health.

The importance of detox smoothies

In the context of Dr. Sebi's method, detox smoothies play a crucial role as they provide an easy and tasty way to eat alkalizing foods. Thanks to their fluid consistency, they promote rapid absorption of nutrients and help reduce the toxin load, facilitating the purification of the body.

To obtain genuinely beneficial smoothies, it is essential to focus on organic fruit and vegetables to avoid the intake of pesticides and chemicals that could compromise the body's purification processes. Minerals- and antioxidant-rich varieties, such as leafy greens (spinach, kale, Swiss chard), cucumbers, berries, and avocados, offer high-level nutritional support: green leaves help maintain an alkaline environment, cucumbers promote hydration thanks to their high-water content. In contrast, berries provide potent antioxidants that can counteract free radicals. Avocado, rich in healthy fats, helps to convey fat-soluble vitamins and make the texture of the smoothie creamier.

A further added value comes from using herbs and spices, such as ginger and turmeric, who's anti-inflammatory and antioxidant properties support the immune system and promote the entire body's well-being. Thanks to its active compounds (gingerols), ginger can help improve digestion and soothe any gastrointestinal discomfort. In contrast, curcumin – the active ingredient in turmeric – helps regulate the inflammatory response and protect cells from oxidative stress.

To complete the recipe, adding oilseeds such as flax and chia enriches the smoothie with essential fatty acids (Omega-3 and Omega-6) and fiber, which support proper intestinal function, helping to reduce inflammation and control cholesterol levels. These seeds also create a "gelling" effect when put in contact with liquids, increasing the sense of satiety and improving the final consistency of the drink. In this way, every sip of the smoothie becomes a concentration of nutrients that work in synergy to promote the balance and vitality of the body.

The choice of ingredients and their combination should balance flavors and nutrients. Mixing low-sugar fruit (to limit glycemic peaks) with green leafy vegetables and superfoods such as spirulina or chlorella allows you to obtain smoothies with a strong detoxifying power and a richness in vitamins, minerals, and vegetable proteins. This holistic approach ensures optimal support for the body, promoting vitality and energy entirely naturally.

Smoothie recipes to detoxify the liver, intestines, and blood

Some smoothie recipes are formulated to support the main organs responsible for purification – liver, intestine, and blood – and promote deep detoxification. Each recipe can be adapted to your tastes, with slightly varying quantities, or by adding your favorite spices and herbs.

1. "Deep Green" Smoothie (Liver)

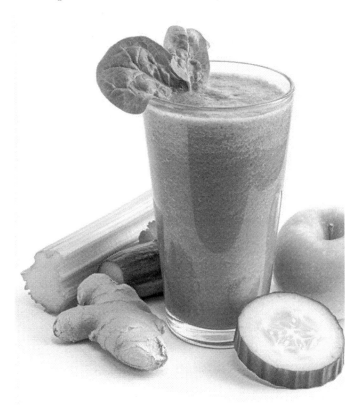

Ingredients:

- 1 cup fresh spinach
- 1/2 cucumber
- 1 stalk of celery
- 1/2 green apple
- Juice of 1/2 lemon
- 1 teaspoon grated ginger (fresh)
- 1 glass of water or coconut water (adjust the amount according to the desired consistency)

Key benefits:

- Spinach, rich in chlorophyll, promotes liver purification.
- Celery and cucumber support hydration and the elimination of toxins.
- Lemon juice and ginger help stimulate liver function.

2. "Detox Swiss Chard" Smoothie (Blood)

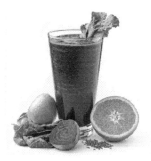

Ingredients:

- 1 small red beetroot (raw or lightly cooked)
- 1 carrot
- 1 peeled orange
- 1 handful of chard leaves (or spinach)
- 1 tsp flaxseed
- Water to taste (or extra carrot juice for fluidizing)

Key benefits:

Beetroot is known to promote blood purification and support the production of red blood cells.

3. "Light Belly" Smoothie (Intestines)

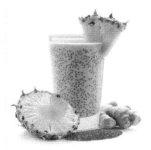

Ingredients:

- 1 cup fresh pineapple
- 1 cup romaine lettuce leaves
- 1 tablespoon chia seeds (soaked for 10 minutes)
- 1 piece of ginger
- 1 teaspoon lemon juice
- Water or coconut water to taste

Key benefits:

Pineapple contains bromelain, an enzyme that aids digestion and helps reduce intestinal inflammation.

4. Artichoke & Lemon Smoothie (Liver & Gallbladder)

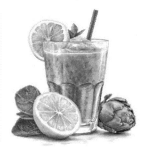

Ingredients:

- 1 cup of already cooked artichoke hearts (preferably steamed)
- 1 handful of arugulas
- Juice of 1 lemon
- 1/2 green apple
- 1 teaspoon of extra virgin olive oil
- Water to taste

Key benefits:

- Artichoke stimulates bile production, facilitating fat digestion and supporting liver function.
- Arugula provides sulfur compounds and chlorophyll for deeper purification.

5. "Fresh & Detoxifying" Smoothie (Blood & Intestines)

Ingredients:

- 1 cup watermelon (or cantaloupe depending on the season)
- 1 cucumber
- 5-6 fresh mint leaves
- 1 teaspoon of hemp seeds (or flax seeds)
- Water to taste

Key benefits:

- Watermelon (or melon) helps hydration and diuresis, promoting the elimination of waste.
- Mint supports digestion and refreshes, helping to reduce any swelling.
- Hemp seeds provide vegetable proteins and fats essential for cellular well-being.

6. Smoothie "Ginger & Turmeric" (Global Anti-Inflammatory)

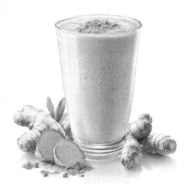

Ingredients:

- 1 cup plant-based milk (almond, oat, or coconut)
- 1 ripe banana
- 1 teaspoon turmeric powder (or a small piece of fresh root)
- 1 piece of fresh ginger
- 1 teaspoon honey (optional) or date for sweetening
- 1 pinch of black pepper (to improve curcumin absorption)

Key benefits:

- Turmeric and ginger have strong anti-inflammatory and antioxidant properties, useful for the liver and immune system.
- Black pepper increases the bioavailability of curcumin.
- Banana and plant-based milk provide creaminess and ready-to-use energy.

7. "LeafGreen" Smoothie (Intestine and Liver)

Ingredients:

- 1 cup kale or spinach
- 1 ripe pear
- 1/2 avocado
- 1 tablespoon lime juice
- 1 teaspoon pumpkin seeds (rich in zinc)
- Water to taste

Key benefits:

- Kale or spinach are sources of chlorophyll and minerals that promote liver detoxification.
- Avocado provides monounsaturated fats and supports the absorption of fat-soluble nutrients.
- Pumpkin seeds, rich in zinc, support the immune system and intestinal health.

1. Smoothie "Ginger & Cucumber" (Purification and Hydration)

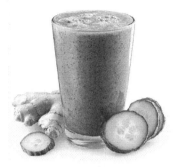

Ingredients:

- 1 medium cucumber
- 1 cup fresh spinach
- 1 piece of fresh ginger (1-2 cm)
- 1 green apple (optional for light sweetening)
- Juice of 1/2 lemon
- Water or coconut water to taste

Key benefits:

- Cucumber and spinach promote diuresis and the elimination of toxins.
- Ginger helps stimulate digestion and reduce inflammation.
- Lemon juice has an alkalizing effect and supports liver function.

2. "Green Apple & Parsley" Smoothie (Immune Booster)

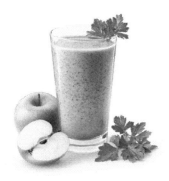

Ingredients:

- 1 green apple
- 1 handful of fresh parsley
- 1 handful of arugulas
- 1 teaspoon chia seeds
- 1/2 glass of natural apple juice (or water)
- 1 teaspoon lime juice

Key benefits:

- Parsley and arugula are rich in chlorophyll and antioxidant substances, useful for purification and immune support.
- The green apple adds fiber and pectin, promoting intestinal regularity.
- Chia seeds provide essential fats and increase the sense of satiety.

3. Orange, Carrot & Turmeric Smoothie (Antioxidant)

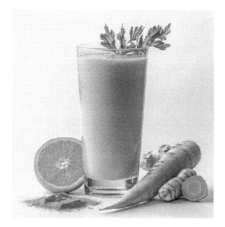

Ingredients:

- 1 peeled orange
- 1 medium carrot
- 1 teaspoon turmeric powder (or a small piece of fresh root)
- 1 piece of fresh ginger (optional)
- 1 pinch of black pepper (to help absorb curcumin
- Water to taste

Key benefits:

- Orange and carrot are rich in beta-carotene and vitamin C, which support the immune system.
- Turmeric and ginger offer anti-inflammatory and antioxidant properties.
- Black pepper increases the bioavailability of curcumin.

4. "Grapefruit & Goji Berries" Smoothie (Metabolism & Fat Burning)

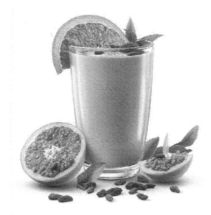

Ingredients:

- 1 peeled pink grapefruit (seeded)
- 1 tablespoon of soaked goji berries
- 1 handful of spinach or kale
- 1 tsp flaxseed
- 1/2 glass of water

Key benefits:

- Grapefruit is known to help regulate fat metabolism.
- Goji berries, rich in antioxidants, support liver and immune function.
- Spinach and flaxseed improve the intake of minerals and fiber.

5. Smoothie "Strawberry, Basil & Flaxseed" (Vascular Protection)

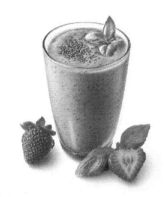

Ingredients:

- 1 cup fresh strawberries
- 4-5 basil leaves
- 1 tablespoon ground flaxseed
- 1/2 cup plant-based milk (almond, rice, or oats)
- 1 teaspoon of honey (optional)

Key benefits:

- Strawberries contain antioxidants that protect blood vessels and cells.
- Basil provides aromatic compounds useful for reducing inflammation and improving digestion.
- Flaxseed provides Omega-3 and supports bowel regularity.

6. "Melon, Mint & Ginger" Smoothie (Freshness and Digestion)

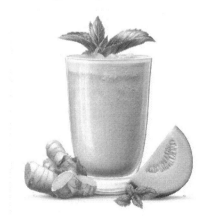

Ingredients:

- 1 cup melon (variety to taste)
- 5-6 fresh mint leaves
- 1 piece of ginger
- 1 teaspoon lemon juice
- Water to taste

Key benefits:

- Melon hydrates and supports diuresis, contributing to the elimination of toxins.
- Mint and ginger help digestion and refresh the gastrointestinal system.
- Lemon offers an alkalizing note and helps preserve vitamin C.

7. "Cherries, Spinach & Chia" Smoothie (Rich in Iron and Antioxidants)

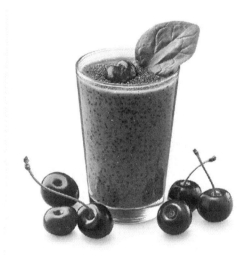

Ingredients:

- 1 cup pitted cherries
- 1 handful of spinach
- 1 tablespoon chia seeds (soaked)
- 1/2 banana for sweetening (optional)
- 1/2 glass of water or vegetable milk

Key benefits:

- Cherries are known for their antioxidant action and melatonin content, which is useful for promoting rest.
- Spinach provides iron and folic acid, which are essential to produce red blood cells.
- Chia seeds improve the intake of fiber and essential fats.

8. "Broccoli, Avocado & Lemon" Smoothie (Vitamins and Minerals)

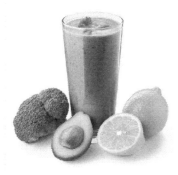

Ingredients:

- 1 cup broccoli florets (lightly blanched or raw, depending on tolerance)
- 1/2 avocado
- Juice of 1/2 lemon
- 1/2 cup water
- 1 teaspoon of extra virgin olive oil (optional)

Key benefits:

- Broccoli contains sulforaphane and antioxidants that promote liver detoxification.
- Avocado, rich in good fats, helps the absorption of fat-soluble vitamins.
- Lemon juice helps maintain a more alkaline pH and supports liver function.

9. "Pear, Banana, Cinnamon & Sunflower Seeds" Smoothie (Sweetness and Energy)

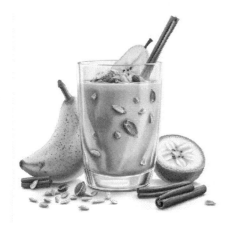

Ingredients:

- 1 ripe pear
- 1 banana
- 1 teaspoon ground cinnamon
- 1 tablespoon of sunflower seeds
- Vegetable milk or water to taste

Key benefits:

- The pear, rich in fiber, promotes intestinal regularity.
- Cinnamon helps balance blood sugar levels and possesses anti-inflammatory properties.
- Sunflower seeds provide B vitamins and vitamin E, which are essential for cellular health.

10. Smoothie "Grape, Fennel & Poppy Seeds" (Draining and Digesting)

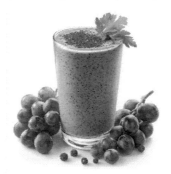

Ingredients:

- 1 cup grapes (preferably red or black, richer in anthocyanins)
- 1/2 fennel
- 1 teaspoon of poppy seeds
- 1 handful lettuce leaves (optional)
- Water to taste

Key benefits:

- Grapes, thanks to anthocyanins, support circulation and offer an antioxidant effect.
- Fennel promotes digestion and helps reduce abdominal bloating.
- Poppy seeds provide calcium and other minerals, supporting healthy bones and muscles.

Final tips for an optimal experience:

- **Immediate preparation:** Consume freshly blended smoothies to avoid nutrient oxidation.
- **Experimentation:** Try different combinations of fruits, vegetables, and spices to find the ideal blend in terms of flavor and benefits.
- **Sugar moderation:** If you prefer a sweeter taste, opt for naturally sugary fruits (banana, mango, dates) in moderate amounts, so as not to overload the glycemic load.

Energizing and anti-inflammatory smoothies

Here is a selection of smoothies designed specifically to provide a boost of energy and, at the same time, help keep inflammatory processes in the body under control. Each recipe can be customized according to everyone's personal preferences or nutritional needs.

1. Smoothie "Chlorophyll Charge"

Ingredients:

- 1 cup fresh spinach
- 1 stalk of celery
- 1/2 avocado
- 1 teaspoon lemon juice
- 1 piece of fresh ginger
- Water or coconut water to taste

Strengths:

- Spinach and celery provide chlorophyll and minerals that improve cell viability.
- Avocado provides healthy fats that promote feelings of satiety and energy stability.
- Ginger has an anti-inflammatory effect and helps to support the immune system.

2. Smoothie "Tropical Boost"

Ingredients:

- 1 cup fresh pineapple
- 1 ripe banana
- 1 tablespoon ground flaxseed
- 1 teaspoon turmeric powder (or a small piece of fresh root)
- 1 pinch of black pepper (to improve curcumin absorption)
- Vegetable milk to taste (almond, oats or coconut)

Strengths:

- Pineapple and banana provide natural sugars and minerals, perfect for a quick energy boost.
- Turmeric acts as a natural anti-inflammatory, assisted by black pepper which enhances its effectiveness.
- Flaxseeds add Omega-3 and fiber, useful for intestinal regularity.

3. "Red Antioxidant" Smoothie

Ingredients:

- 1 cup mixed berries (blueberries, raspberries, blackberries)
- 1 small beetroot (raw or lightly cooked)
- 1 teaspoon chia seeds
- 1 date (optional, for sweetening)
- Water or coconut water to taste

Strengths:

- Berries are rich in anthocyanins, powerful antioxidants that fight oxidative stress.
- Beetroot supports circulation and the production of red blood cells, contributing to tissue oxygenation.
- Chia seeds provide long-term energy and promote the stability of blood sugar levels.

4. "Zen Turmeric & Mango" Smoothie

Ingredients:

- 1 cup ripe mango
- 1 teaspoon turmeric powder (or a small piece of fresh root)
- 1 piece of ginger

- 1/2 teaspoon coconut oil (optional, improves curcumin absorption)
- Vegetable milk to taste

Strengths:

- Mango, rich in vitamin C and beta-carotene, provides energy and promotes healthy skin.
- Turmeric and ginger act synergistically as anti-inflammatory and digestive.
- Coconut oil helps to make the fat-soluble active ingredients in turmeric more bioavailable.

5. "Vegetable Protein" Smoothie

Ingredients:

- 1 handful of kale leaves or spinach
- 1 banana
- 1 tablespoon almond butter or sunflower seed butter
- 1 teaspoon hemp seeds (rich in protein)
- Vegetable milk to taste

Strengths:

- Kale and spinach provide chlorophyll, iron, and minerals for healthy blood oxygenation.
- Almond butter and hemp seeds are sources of protein and essential fats, great for prolonged energy.
- The high micronutrient content supports repair processes and reduces inflammation.

6. Smoothie "Avocado & Spirulina"

Ingredients:

- 1/2 avocado
- 1 teaspoon of spirulina powder
- 1 handful of spinach or lettuce
- 1/2 green apple (optional for sweetening)
- Water or coconut water to taste

Strengths:

- Spirulina is an algae rich in proteins, vitamins and minerals, known for its antioxidant action.
- Avocado provides monounsaturated fats that support cardiovascular well-being and nutrient absorption.
- The green leaves complete the picture of micronutrients and chlorophyll, promoting detoxification.

7. Grapefruit & Mint Smoothie

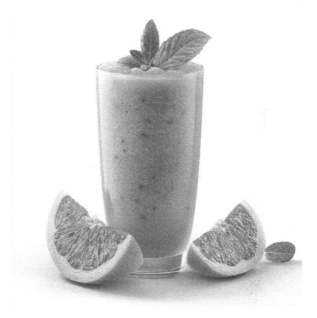

Ingredients:

- 1 pink grapefruit (raw peeled)
- 5-6 fresh mint leaves
- 1 tsp flaxseed
- 1/2 cucumber
- 1 piece of ginger (optional)
- Water to taste

Strengths:

- Grapefruit helps stimulate metabolism and provides a supply of vitamin C.
- Fresh mint promotes digestion and gives a feeling of freshness.
- Flaxseed enriches the mix of essential fatty acids, improving the overall anti-inflammatory effect.

8. Chocolate & Cayenne Smoothie

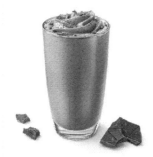

Ingredients:

- 1 tablespoon of unsweetened cocoa powder (organic)
- 1 banana
- 1 pinch of cayenne pepper
- 1 teaspoon peanut butter (optional)
- Vegetable milk to taste

Strengths:

- Unsweetened cocoa is rich in antioxidant flavonoids, which are useful for cardiovascular health and inflammation reduction.
- Cayenne pepper can boost metabolism and promote circulation.
- The addition of peanut butter increases protein and energy intake.

9. Peach & Ginger Smoothie

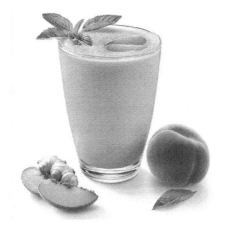

Ingredients:

- 2 ripe peaches (or nectarines)
- 1 piece of fresh ginger
- 1 handful of lettuce leaves
- 1 teaspoon of hemp seeds
- Water or coconut water to taste

Strengths:

- Peaches provide vitamins and antioxidants, as well as a natural sweet flavor.
- Ginger enhances the anti-inflammatory effect and promotes digestion.
- Hemp seeds add high-quality protein and essential fats.

10. Banana & Cinnamon Smoothie

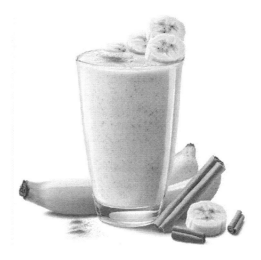

Ingredients:

- 1 ripe banana
- 1 teaspoon ground cinnamon
- 1 teaspoon chia seeds (soaked)
- 1 handful arugula (optional for a slightly spicy touch)
- Vegetable milk (almond, oat or coconut) to taste

Strengths:

- The banana provides potassium, useful for regulating blood pressure and supporting muscle contraction.
- Cinnamon helps stabilize blood sugar levels and possesses anti-inflammatory properties.
- Chia seeds contribute to better blood sugar control and offer Omega-3 fatty acids.

CHAPTER 22: DR. SEBI HERB'S ENCYCLOPEDIA – THE ENCYCLOPEDIA OF HEALING HERBS

Dr. Sebi's history is deeply linked to the constant search for natural solutions that can support and restore the balance of the body. From first-hand observations of the benefits of wild herbs in his native Honduras, Dr. Sebi developed the belief that many diseases could be prevented and cured by returning the body to an alkaline state, in which toxins and excess mucus were gradually eliminated. Over the years, he deepened his knowledge of medicinal plants, experimenting with herbal remedies capable of detoxifying the body and strengthening the immune system.

This "Encyclopedia of Healing Herbs" represents the essence of that research: a journey through the treasures of phytotherapy, according to Dr. Sebi, where each herb is analyzed for its specific properties and the role it can play in maintaining or recovering health. The common thread is that an alkaline body, nourished by high-quality phytochemicals, is the prerequisite for a strong and responsive immune system. Although times and contexts have changed, Dr. Sebi's original intuition retains all its strength today, offering ideas for a natural medicine rooted in the ancient wisdom of plants.

In this chapter, we'll explore the most potent alkaline herbs and their benefits and explain how to choose and use each one based on individual needs. We will then delve into the drying and preservation techniques and the different preparation methods: herbal teas, decoctions, tinctures, and compresses. Finally, according to Dr. Sebi, a complete guide to phytotherapy will be offered, with particular attention to the most effective detox herbs to purify the liver, kidneys, and blood in compliance with a holistic approach that integrates nutrition, lifestyle, and natural practices. The richness of this chapter lies in the union between traditional wisdom and Dr. Sebi's empirical experience: it is not simply a list of herbs but an invitation to rediscover the power of nature as a precious ally in the pursuit of well-being. Each herb tells a story of therapeutic properties, synergies with other plants, and often underestimated potential. Knowing and applying this knowledge correctly means putting in one's hands the possibility of acting proactively on health through simple gestures that respect the body.

The herbs of Honduras

The cultural roots of medicinal herbs go back to ancient times, and, in the specific case of Dr. Sebi, they draw lifebloods mainly from the traditions of Honduras and other Mesoamerican cultures. Honduras, located in the heart of Central America, represents a crossroads of peoples and knowledge: over the centuries, different indigenous ethnic groups have met here, such as the Lenca, the Pech, and the Garifuna, who have handed down from generation to generation an in-depth knowledge of local plants and their healing properties.

Over the centuries, the indigenous communities of Honduras have developed a symbiotic relationship with the surrounding environment. Rainforests, plateaus, and coastal areas offer an incredible variety of plant species. The inhabitants of these regions learned to recognize and catalog medicinal plants, experimenting with their effectiveness in treating wounds, infectious diseases, and chronic ailments. Much of this knowledge was passed down orally: it was the healers, the "curanderos," and the elderly women of the village who kept the secrets of how to collect herbs, in which phase of the moon it was preferable to dry them, and with which other plants it was appropriate to combine them to enhance their effectiveness. Mesoamerica, a historical region that includes today's southern Mexico, Guatemala, Belize, El Salvador, and Honduras, was the cradle of great civilizations such as the Mayans and Aztecs. These people had developed a complex system of herbal knowledge based on a cosmic and spiritual vision of health. For the Maya, for example, the human body was part of a larger sacred order. Plants served to heal physical diseases and restore harmony between the individual and the universe. Although partly lost, the Mayan codices contain references to plants that treat fevers, infections, digestive disorders, and even spiritual and divinatory rituals.

Similarly, Aztec tradition boasted royal botanical gardens with medicinal plants from all over the empire. The Aztecs had a very advanced medical system for the time, with figures of "city" (healers) specialized in preparing ointments, poultices, and herbal drinks. Again, healing was a holistic process involving body, mind, and spirit.

Growing up in Honduras, Dr. Sebi absorbed these traditions in a natural way: medicinal plants and folk remedies were part of the daily life of many rural communities. Observing how the locals treated themselves with root decoctions, leaf compresses, and tropical fruit juices, he developed the conviction that nature offered practical answers to most human health problems. So he began to experiment and catalog the area's plants, drawing inspiration from local knowledge and a much older Mesoamerican heritage.

Although Dr. Sebi was trained in a Honduran context, his herbal approach was not limited to the country's geographical boundaries. Over time, he expanded his research by studying plants from various parts of the world, comparing the properties of African, South American, and Asian herbs. This cultural and herbal syncretism allowed him to build a unique method that combined the philosophy of the alkaline diet with a solid phytotherapeutic basis. However, the intuition behind his work remained the one he had learned in Honduras: a body in harmony with nature, nourished by authentic and uncontaminated plants, possesses an extraordinary capacity for self-healing.

Although much of the knowledge originating in Mesoamerican cultures is in danger of being lost, Dr. Sebi's contribution shows how precious and relevant it is. Today, the rediscovery of ancient texts and field research in indigenous communities make it possible to recover part of this knowledge, putting it at the service of modern phytotherapy, attentive to effectiveness and respect for natural cycles. Many herbs Dr.

Sebi recommended – such as sarsaparilla, burdock, nettle, or dandelion – have their roots in a thousand-year-old tradition, shared by peoples far away in space but close in recognizing the power of nature.

The cultural origins of the medicinal herbs that inspired Dr. Sebi demonstrate how popular wisdom, often passed down orally, can offer valuable insights for a holistic approach to health. Honduras and Mesoamerica represent, in this sense, a crossroads of civilizations that have been able to dialogue with nature and understand its secrets. Dr. Sebi's work is part of this legacy: he recovers and modernizes these traditions, integrating them with the needs of contemporary life. Choosing to use medicinal plants is a gesture of care for one's body and a way to honor those peoples' history and reconnect to a dimension of respect and harmony with the earth.

The Most Powerful Alkaline Herbs and Their Benefits

Alkaline herbs are a key component of Dr. Sebi's method, who argued that maintaining a mildly alkaline internal environment was crucial to promoting the body's self-healing. According to this view, many diseases originate from an excess of acidity and consequent inflammation; therefore, introducing alkaline medicinal plants can help rebalance the pH, supporting purification processes and boosting the immune system.

Alkaline herbs are characterized by their ability to help keep the body's pH in an optimal range (slightly above 7). On a practical level, no "universal table" accurately lists the pH value of each plant. However, experience and empirical research have made it possible to identify some herbs known for their alkalizing effects. These plants generally have a high concentration of minerals such as calcium, magnesium, and potassium and contain phytochemical compounds that counteract systemic acidity. On the contrary, herbs or acidic foods promote mucus formation and overload the excretory organs.

1. Nettle (Urtica dioica)

According to Dr. Sebi, nettle is considered an alkaline herb capable of supporting overall well-being due to its high content of minerals such as iron, silicon, and calcium. Nettle endorses the elimination of nitrogenous waste and promotes kidney function, thus helping to maintain a clean indoor environment free of toxic accumulations. In the context of Dr. Sebi's encyclopedia, nettle is often referred to as an "electric food" for its energizing and remineralizing power. It can be taken as herbal tea, decoction, or mother tincture. It is particularly suitable for those who want to reduce inflammation and improve circulation.

2. Burdock (Arctium lappa)

Burdock is one of the herbs most cited by Dr. Sebi for its strong purifying properties. Rich in inulin and anti-inflammatory compounds, it acts on the liver and kidneys, helping to remove toxins from the blood and supporting the lymphatic system. In Dr. Sebi's vision, impurity-free blood circulation prevents skin disorders such as eczema or psoriasis. Burdock can be taken as herbal tea (using the dried root), mother tincture, or tablets. The root boiled for a long time (15-20 minutes) releases its active ingredients effectively, promoting tissue regeneration and reducing skin inflammation.

3. Sarsaparilla (Smilax ornata)

Sarsaparilla, which Dr. Sebi considers very valuable, is known for its ability to purify the blood and support kidney function. Rich in saponins, it helps eliminate metabolic residues and pathogens that can circulate in the body, counteracting infections and inflammation. According to Dr. Sebi's phytotherapeutic encyclopedia, sarsaparilla is particularly useful for people who want to lighten the load of toxins on the body, facilitating diuresis and lymphatic drainage. It can be prepared in decoction by boiling the root for 10-15 minutes or as a dry extract, to be taken in capsules or powder.

4. Dandelion (Taraxacum officinale)

Dandelion, prized for its beneficial effect on the liver and digestive system, is cited by Dr. Sebi as one of the most effective herbs for maintaining pH balance. Thanks to its purifying properties, it promotes bile production and contributes to a more active metabolism. The leaves, rich in vitamins and minerals, can be added raw to salads. At the same time, the root is used to prepare herbal teas or decoctions that stimulate liver function. In Dr. Sebi's philosophy, a healthy liver is the basis of an organism capable of defending itself against inflammatory states and recovering energy faster.

5. Licorice root (Glycyrrhiza glabra)

Licorice root, in addition to being known for its characteristic sweet taste, plays a particular role in Dr. Sebi's approach due to its antiviral and immunomodulatory properties. It helps support the adrenal glands, which is helpful in chronic stress or fatigue. According to Dr. Sebi, licorice's ability to soothe mucous membranes and regulate cortisol levels helps maintain a more alkaline internal environment less prone to inflammatory processes. It is recommended to use it in moderation in case of hypertension, as it can raise blood pressure. Generally, the root is taken as herbal tea (leaving the pieces to infuse for 10 minutes) or in powder form added to smoothies or culinary preparations.

6. Fucus seaweed (Fucus vesiculosus)

Although it is not a terrestrial herb, Dr. Sebi often focuses on lists of foods and natural remedies due to its high content of iodine, minerals, and essential trace elements. It helps regulate thyroid function, stimulstimulatelism, and contrimanageeight. According to Dr. Sebi's approach, a correct hormonal balance also passes through an adequate intake of iodine, which promotes the production of thyroid hormones and the purification of heavy metals in the body. Fucus can be taken in herbal tea, capsules, or powder, with attention to the dosage, especially in the presence of thyroid diseases.

Each of these herbs, according to Dr. Sebi's encyclopedia and approach, works synergistically with the body's self-healing processes, helping to create a more alkaline, less prone to inflammation, and more energy-efficient internal environment. Choosing the right plant, based on specific needs, and taking it consistently, allows you to fully exploit the potential of each remedy, integrating it into a wellness path that includes healthy eating, adequate hydration, and balanced lifestyles.

Key health benefits

Alkaline herbs offer numerous health benefits, helping to cleanse the blood and excretory organs, reduce chronic inflammation, regulate internal pH, and support the immune system due to their rich content of minerals and herbal compounds. According to Dr. Sebi's philosophy, these plants are essential because the human body is designed to function at its best in an environment free of excess mucus and characterized by a slightly alkaline pH. By choosing plants that are not hybridized and rich in active ingredients, Dr. Sebi aimed to restore the body's natural chemical-physical balance, laying the foundation for optimal health and increased resistance to infection.

Gradually introducing alkaline herbs into your diet is essential to allow the body to gently and safely adapt to the new active ingredients, avoiding adverse reactions and fully appreciating the benefits of each individual plant. A progressive, rather than intensive, approach allows you to assess your personal tolerance and integrate herbs into your daily routine in a balanced way. For example, you can start with one cup a day of a light infusion, such as nettle or dandelion, to gradually accustom your palate and monitor your body's responses. For those short on time or who prefer a more immediate supplementation method, dry extracts in capsule or powder form are an excellent solution, as they can be easily added to smoothies, soups, or other preparations. In addition, some herbs, such as nettle or dandelion, can be incorporated directly into daily meals, such as salads, soups, sauces, or omelets, to enrich the diet with minerals and beneficial substances without significantly altering the flavor. Finally, alternating the different herbs during the week is a valuable strategy to vary the nutritional profile and reduce the risk of intolerances, ensuring a broader intake of active ingredients and enhancing the overall benefits for the body.

The most potent alkaline herbs, at the heart of Dr. Sebi's approach, are essential contributors to maintaining pH balance and promoting robust health. They help the body cleanse itself, reduce inflammation, and strengthen the immune system, creating the ideal environment for the activation of self-healing mechanisms. Gradually integrating these plants into your daily diet—whether herbal teas, extracts, or simple recipes—allows you to experience their effects in a safe and sustainable way, promoting a lifestyle in harmony with nature.

Role of Minerals in Alkaline Herbs and Their Impact on the Body's pH

The minerals found in alkaline herbs – such as calcium, magnesium, iron, and potassium – play a key role in maintaining a slightly alkaline body pH. As chemical "buffers," they help neutralize excess acidity generated by stress, improper nutrition, or inflammatory processes. According to Dr. Sebi, this balance is essential to allow the body to perform its functions at its best, from enzymatic reactions to tissue regeneration. A body in which the pH remains alkaline tends to reduce the accumulation of mucus and counteract the proliferation of pathogens, promoting an internal environment in which the immune defenses are more effective and self-healing processes can be activated more quickly.

Extraction techniques and concentration of active ingredients

The extraction and concentration techniques of active ingredients in medicinal plants aim to obtain preparations in which the beneficial substances are present in a more concentrated form that is easily assimilated by the body. Herbal teas and decoctions represent the most traditional methods: in the first case, the herbs are poured into hot water for a few minutes, an ideal method for delicate flowers and leaves; in the second, the woody parts or roots are boiled for a longer time, thus releasing more resistant compounds. On the other hand, mother tinctures involve a prolonged maceration of the herbs in alcohol or glycerin for a few weeks, obtaining a liquid with a high concentration of active ingredients in drops, allowing precise dosing. A further approach is an extraction with natural solvents, such as oil or glycerine, used to make oolites or glycerine extracts, which preserve the original phytocomplex profile. These techniques, if carried out with attention to the ideal times and temperatures, not only enhance the therapeutic properties of the plants but also allow for better preservation of the active ingredients, facilitating their absorption and long-term effectiveness.

Customise phytotherapy according to your biological constitution

Customizing phytotherapy according to one's biological constitution means recognizing that everyone has unique needs and that medicinal herbs can be selected and dosed to harmonize with one's physiological and metabolic profile. This strategy begins with carefully analyzing one's constitution, including assessments of energy levels, digestion, sensitivity to inflammation, and hormonal balance. It is essential, for example, to consider whether you are predisposed to a more acidic or alkaline state, experience symptoms of chronic fatigue or stress, or your immune system is susceptible to external factors. Once these characteristics have been identified, herbs can be chosen that act in synergy with specific needs: for those who need more purification, herbs such as dandelion or dandelion can be opted for, while to support energy and reduce stress, adaptogenic herbs such as ashwagandha or ginseng may be the most suitable. A personalized approach also includes combining different preparation methods – for example, herbal teas for the gradual absorption of active ingredients and tinctures for a more concentrated effect – and varying the frequency and dosage according to the body's responses. In this way, phytotherapy does not become a universal remedy but a tailor-made path that dynamically adapts to individual needs, offering constant support to improve well-being and prevent the occurrence of imbalances.

How to choose and use herbs for specific treatments

Hypertension can be addressed with nettle (Urtica dioica), a plant rich in minerals such as calcium and magnesium. It helps regulate blood pressure and improve circulation. Thanks to its diuretic properties, it promotes the elimination of excess fluids, lightening the load on the cardiovascular system. It can be taken as herbal tea (one or two cups daily) or a capsule dry extract.

Dandelion (Taraxacum officinale) is particularly indicated for digestive and gastric disorders. This plant supports liver and biliary function, promoting bile production and helping to regulate digestive processes. Its purifying effect helps to reduce acidity and inflammation in the stomach. Dandelion can be used as a root decoction (boiled in water for ten to fifteen minutes) or by adding fresh leaves to salads.

Burdock (Arctium lappa) is often recommended for skin diseases such as eczema and psoriasis. Known for its purifying and anti-inflammatory properties, it acts on the liver and blood, helping to eliminate toxins that can occur in the skin. It also promotes tissue regeneration and reduces itching. It is generally taken as herbal tea or mother tincture, with a certain constancy (at least three to four weeks).

Sarsaparilla (Smilax ornata) is an effective option for urinary tract infections. Rich in saponins and anti-inflammatory compounds, it promotes blood purification and supports kidney function, helping the body fight bacterial infections. Its diuretic action "washes away" pathogens and can be exploited through infusion or decoction. It must be taken once or twice a day, accompanied by adequate hydration.

When suffering from chronic fatigue and stress, licorice root (Glycyrrhiza glabra) offers valuable support. In addition to possessing antiviral properties, it acts as an adrenal tonic, supporting the body's response to stress. It helps balance cortisol levels and provides a mild energizing effect without using synthetic stimulants. You can prepare an herbal tea with small pieces of root, infusing them for ten minutes or adding the powder to smoothies. However, it is essential to use it in moderation in case of hypertension, as licorice can raise it even further.

For those suffering from arthritis and joint pain, ginger (Zingiber officinale) is a natural ally. Its gingerols have powerful anti-inflammatory properties, helping to reduce joint pain and stiffness. It also stimulates circulation and promotes the drainage of toxins related to inflammatory processes. Ginger is taken in the form of herbal tea (grated or sliced fresh ginger) or as a powder added to hot dishes or smoothies.

Conversely, if excess mucus and bronchitis are a problem, thyme (Thymus vulgaris) can offer valuable help. Thanks to its high antiseptic and mucolytic activity, it promotes the expulsion of excess mucus and counteracts bacterial proliferation. It is indicated for respiratory health, helping to soothe coughs and irritation. An infusion of thyme (a teaspoon of leaves dried in hot water for ten minutes) can be taken twice to three times a day or used as a fume component.

Lavender (Lavandula angustifolia) is particularly suitable for recurrent headaches, as it relaxes the nervous system and has mild analgesic properties. It helps calm states of tension and reduce the frequency and intensity of headaches of muscle tension or stress-related origin. You can prepare an infusion of lavender flowers (one teaspoon per cup of water) to sip in a quiet environment or diffuse a few drops of essential oil.

Sage (Salvia officinalis) offers valuable support for menstrual disorders and premenstrual syndrome (PMS). It contains phytoestrogens and essential oils that help regulate hormonal balance, reducing menstrual pain, bloating, and mood swings. Sage can be taken as herbal tea (a teaspoon of dried leaves in boiling water for five to seven minutes) once or twice a day, especially before or during the cycle.

Rashes and skin allergies can benefit red clover (Trifolium pratense). Thanks to its cleansing and anti-inflammatory properties, it supports skin health. It relieves symptoms such as itching, redness, or rashes. In addition, its hormonally balancing action can be helpful in allergic reactions related to internal imbalances. It can be taken as an infusion of flowers (one to two teaspoons in hot water for ten minutes), to be drunk once or twice a day, or applied topically in the form of a compress to soothe skin irritations.

The choice of the most suitable herb depends on the nature of the ailment, individual constitution, and general state of health. A holistic approach – including a balanced diet, adequate hydration, and a healthy lifestyle – enhances the effectiveness of alkaline herbs. The important thing is to proceed gradually and monitor your body's reactions, possibly seeking advice from an experienced phytotherapy professional to obtain lasting results and complete safety.

Phytotherapy and prevention

Phytotherapy, when consistently integrated into everyday life, can play a decisive role in preventing relapses or worsening of existing disorders. Regularly using herbs with immunomodulating, purifying, or anti-inflammatory properties – think nettle for circulation, dandelion for liver function, licorice for adrenal stress – creates a more stable "biological ground" in which the body's natural defenses are always ready to intervene. However, it is essential to proceed gradually, perhaps starting with a single herbal tea daily and then increasing the frequency or variety of plants used to allow the body to adapt without stress. In addition, adopting periodic cycles – for example, dedicating a few weeks to a specific herb, then switching to another – helps to avoid addiction to the active ingredients and vary the range of beneficial substances.

To best maintain preventive effectiveness, combining phytotherapy with a balanced diet rich in fresh and whole foods and a lifestyle that includes physical movement and stress management techniques is advisable. In this way, herbs do not become a simple remedy to be taken in an emergency. Still, continuous support keeps the body balanced, significantly reducing the risk of flare-ups and ensuring longer-lasting well-being.

Techniques for drying, storing, and preparing herbs

Knowing the correct techniques for drying, storing, and preparing herbs is essential to preserve their therapeutic properties as much as possible. Medicinal plants, in fact, are rich in active ingredients – including essential oils, flavonoids, and polyphenols – which are extremely sensitive to oxygen, light, and humidity. If handled inappropriately, these valuable components are likely to degrade or evaporate, significantly reducing the beneficial power that weed could offer. Learning to treat plants with care, from harvesting to final preparation, means guaranteeing a high-quality phytotherapeutic remedy, which can be used over time for numerous uses: from daily infusions and decoctions to culinary preparations, up to more complex formulations such as tinctures, ointments or medicated oils.

The correct processing of herbs becomes even more crucial, aiming to maintain an alkaline and toxin-free internal environment. Each step, from plant selection to drying method, significantly impacts the concentration of active ingredients and their bioavailability. For example, an herb that keeps its essential oils intact promotes a better immune response and offers a more pronounced anti-inflammatory effect; on the contrary, rapid drying at high temperatures can irreparably compromise the quality of the final product.

Knowing how to store herbs long-term allows you to build a tiny home "natural pharmacy," ready to use any time of the year. This is particularly useful when you want to maintain a constant wellness routine: having herbal teas and decoctions available to consume regularly, or extracts and powders to add to dishes or smoothies, allows you to integrate the phytotherapeutic properties into everyday life. This ability to "manage" herbs independently, respecting their natural cycles and protecting them from degradation factors, translates into greater control over one's health and a more profound harmony with the rhythms of nature.

Drying Techniques

Air drying is the most natural method. It consists of choosing a dry, shady, and well-ventilated place where the herbs are placed in thin layers on racks or nets, occasionally turning them. This process, which avoids direct contact with sunlight to not degrade the essential oils, is ideal for preserving the active ingredients. Ensure that your plants are clean and free of surface moisture. Alternatively, you can use an oven or dryer by setting the temperature between 30 and 40 °C, constantly monitoring the degree of drying so as not to overheat the leaves. This solution reduces time and offers greater control, especially if you leave the door slightly open in the case of the oven to ensure air exchange. Finally, for plants with long stems, such as lavender, rosemary, and sage, you can opt for drying in hanging bunches: group the herbs in small bunches tied at the base with a string and hang them upside down in a dry and dark place, avoiding humid environments or those subject to excessive drafts; Once dried, the leaves crumble and place in tightly closed containers.

Conservation Techniques

One of the most common solutions to properly store dried herbs to properly store dried herbs is to store them in airtight containers, such as airtight and possibly dark-colored glass jars, to protect them from humidity and oxidation, preserving aromas and active ingredients. Labeling the jars indicating the herb's name and the drying date is also helpful. Another technique consists of a vacuum, where the air is removed from the bags before sealing, significantly extending the shelf life and reducing the risk of contamination by mold or bacteria: it is advisable to periodically check that the bags remain intact. In some cases, you can opt for freezing, particularly for herbs such as parsley or basil, which retain their aroma well if chopped and placed in small containers or food bags in the freezer. It is preferable to thaw only the necessary amount to not compromise the consistency and nutritional qualities of the rest.

Preparation in general

Herbal teas and infusions are made by pouring boiling water over dried herbs (usually 1 teaspoon of herb per cup of water), covering the container, and leaving to infuse for 5-10 minutes. Reserve the essential oils and adjust the desired intensity. Decoctions, on the other hand, are more suitable for roots, bark, and woody parts: boil the herb in water for 10-15 minutes over low heat, then filter, taking care not to prolong the boiling too long so as not to degrade the thermolabile components. The mother tinctures, and extracts are prepared by macerating the herbs in alcohol (or glycerine) for 2-4 weeks in a closed container, then filtering the liquid and storing it in dark glass bottles: the result is a concentrated, practical, and long-life form, to be dosed carefully. Finally, to obtain oils and ointments for topical use, the herbs are left to macerate in a carrier oil (such as olive or almond oil) for several weeks, filtering everything at the end of the process. By adding beeswax, you get ointments with a solid consistency, ideal for applications on the skin and mucous membranes, with soothing, anti-inflammatory, or healing effects depending on the plant chosen.

Complete guide to phytotherapy according to Dr. Sebi

According to Dr. Sebi's approach, phytotherapy is a holistic method that integrates herbs to restore the body's balance and promote self-healing. Dr. Sebi firmly believed that well-being came from a natural diet enriched with non-hybridized herbs capable of keeping the body's internal environment alkaline. His vision was based on the idea that by eliminating toxins and reducing mucus buildup, the body could regain its intrinsic ability to heal and protect, working in synergy with its natural defense mechanisms.

The phytotherapy guide is based on carefully selecting medicinal plants, thoroughly understanding their specific properties, and applying correct preparation and administration techniques. In this context, each herb is chosen not only for its isolated therapeutic effect but also for its ability to interact positively with the immune system and excretory organs, promoting a natural balance that supports overall health. The goal is to transform the simple use of herbal remedies into an authentic lifestyle capable of proactively preventing and counteracting diseases.

A fundamental aspect of this approach concerns the integration of phytotherapy into the daily diet. Combining medicinal herbs with a healthy diet allows you to maximize the benefits derived from the active ingredients present in plants, creating a synergistic effect with natural foods. For example, adding alkaline herbal infusions or decoctions to meals rich in fruits, vegetables, and whole grains can help keep the body's pH in balance, stimulate digestion, and facilitate the elimination of toxins. This constant integration into the dietary routine allows phytotherapy to be used as a continuous support for health and well-being.

The synergy between herbs and nutraceuticals is another key element of Dr. Sebi's method. In this context, the interaction between medicinal herbs, superfoods, and natural supplements significantly boosts the immune system. Herbs, rich in minerals, vitamins, and phytochemicals, work with nutrients found in superfoods, such as berries, algae, and oilseeds, to provide the body with integrated protection against external aggressions. The combined use of these elements makes it possible to create personalized formulas capable of responding to the specific needs of everyone, improving resistance to infections and accelerating cell regeneration processes.

Phytotherapy can be adopted as a preventive strategy to counteract the onset of chronic diseases and infections. Using herbs as a preventive tool means incorporating remedies into your daily routine that, in addition to treating the symptoms, act on the root causes of the disorders. This preventive practice translates into the regular intake of infusions, tinctures, and decoctions that help maintain a strong immune system, reduce inflammation, and support the purifying action of internal organs. By doing so, the body is better equipped to cope with environmental and metabolic stresses, reducing the risk of developing chronic diseases and improving quality of life. Scientific research has provided numerous evidence to support the use of medicinal herbs to improve health, integrating the principles of phytotherapy with modern science. Studies such as those by Arts and Hollman have shown that flavonoids – found in many alkaline herbs – modulate the immune response and protect cells from oxidative stress, helping to reduce inflammation. Similarly, Williamson's research emphasized the importance of synergy between various phytochemicals, demonstrating that the interaction between active plant ingredients can enhance therapeutic effects far beyond individual isolated extracts.

A review published in the Journal of Environmental and Public Health analyzed the impact of a diet rich in alkalizing foods, suggesting that a slightly alkaline indoor environment is crucial for preventing inflammation and metabolic dysfunction. In addition, a systematic study on the role of polyphenols has confirmed their anti-inflammatory and antioxidant properties, which are essential for counteracting chronic diseases and supporting the immune system.

Other studies published in the Journal of Ethnopharmacology and Phytotherapy Research have examined the role of specific herbs – such as dandelion and burdock – in supporting liver function and blood purification, demonstrating how these traditional remedies can help eliminate accumulated toxins. Finally, a meta-analysis on strengthening the immune system through herbal supplements has shown that the constant use of medicinal herbs improves the body's ability to fight infections, significantly boosting the natural defenses.

These studies confirm the effectiveness of herbal remedies and reinforce the idea that a holistic approach – based on alkaline herbs, natural nutrition, and supplementation with nutraceuticals – can be a winning preventive and therapeutic strategy. This scientific evidence represents the bridge between traditional wisdom and modern health needs, making phytotherapy a precious ally for global well-being.

The most effective detox herbs

Detox herbs play a key role in supporting the body's natural cleansing process, helping to eliminate toxins and accumulated waste. Plants such as burdock, dandelion, sarsaparilla, and nettle are among the most used in this area, thanks to their combined action on the liver, kidneys, and lymphatic system. To make the most of the benefits of these herbs, it is essential to choose appropriate preparations: herbal teas and decoctions are particularly effective for roots and leaves. At the same time, tinctures or concentrated extracts can speed up the absorption of active ingredients. It is also advisable to gradually integrate detox herbs into the daily routine and associate them with a diet rich in natural and alkalizing foods to enhance the purifying action and maintain an internal environment conducive to overall well-being.

Combination of Detox Herbs and Functional Foods

Supplementing detox herbs with functional foods – commonly known as superfoods – can significantly enhance the purifying benefits, offering the body a combination of active ingredients that work in synergy. Detox herbs, such as burdock, dandelion, and sarsaparilla, act mainly on the liver, kidneys, and lymphatic system, facilitating the elimination of toxins and metabolic waste. On the other hand, Superfoods are rich in key nutrients such as vitamins, minerals, essential fatty acids, and antioxidants, all of which help restore the body's balance and support immune function. When purifying herbs are combined with foods with high nutritional value (for example, algae such as spirulina or chlorella, oilseeds such as chia or flax, and fruit rich in antioxidants such as berries), a "cascade" effect is created: toxins are mobilized and conveyed to the excretory organs, while the cells receive regenerating support thanks to the presence of essential micronutrients. This synergy is particularly effective in promoting an alkaline internal environment, reducing inflammation, and optimizing metabolic processes.

Through his practice and the numerous testimonies of patients, Dr. Sebi noticed that a diet rich in alkaline herbs and superfoods could significantly accelerate the detoxification phase. He argued that medicinal plants and natural, non-hybridized foods created a "biological soil" favorable to self-healing. This soil, defined by Sebi as free of excess mucus and acidifying substances, was the prerequisite for lasting health, in which the body, thanks to the support of minerals and antioxidants, recovered its vital energy and better-resisted infections.

Herbal teas and smoothies can be creatively combined to intensify the process of eliminating toxins. For example, a purifying herbal tea based on dandelion and nettle can become the basic liquid for a fruit and vegetable smoothie, blending the alkalizing and diuretic properties of herbs with the vitamins and polyphenols of green leafy vegetables, berries, or oilseeds. Similarly, detox herbal powders such as dried burdock root can be added to functional salads, enriched with hemp or pumpkin seeds, to maintain a stable pH and reduce systemic inflammation.

Another strategy is to integrate sarsaparilla decoctions, dandelion, or milk thistle into the cooking of whole grains such as rice, millet, or quinoa, allowing the grains to absorb the active ingredients of the plants. Those who prefer a more concentrated approach can combine algae extracts (spirulina or chlorella) with detox herbal tinctures, thus combining the richness of chlorophyll and trace elements with a concentrate of active ingredients in a quickly assimilable form. It is always advisable to alternate the different herbs and superfoods during the week, avoiding an overload of substances and ensuring a varied intake of nutrients. The gradual introduction of these combinations helps to identify the formula that best suits one's needs, observing how the body responds and adapting the doses in a personalized way.

This synergy between detox herbs and functional foods intensifies purification and offers high-level nutritional support. Dr. Sebi's observations highlight the importance of maintaining an alkaline and inflammation-free body and exploiting the healing potential of medicinal plants and superfoods. With a gradual and conscious approach, in which different combinations are experimented, it is possible to consolidate eating habits that promote lasting vitality and well-being.

Balancing plant-based protein intake

Balancing the intake of vegetable proteins becomes essential when including herbs and superfoods to support a more alkaline or detox diet. Suppose your goal is to reduce your consumption of animal protein. In that case, it is necessary to make sure that your meals include complete protein sources, such as legumes (chickpeas, lentils, beans), whole grains (brown rice, quinoa, spelled), and oilseeds (chia, hemp, pumpkin). Combined, these foods provide the full spectrum of essential amino acids. In addition, many herbs and superfoods help improve the bioavailability of nutrients. For example, adding ginger or spices like chili peppers can promote digestion and protein assimilation. Algae (spirulina, chlorella, nori) is another valuable help, as they are rich in high-quality proteins and micronutrients. Finally, regularly varying plant sources help cover the need for amino acids in a balanced way, avoiding deficiencies and supporting the cleansing properties of herbs simultaneously.

Herb Rotation Strategies

Alternating different types of herbs during the week is a practical approach to optimize the results of a phytotherapeutic path. In fact, each plant has a unique set of active ingredients and minerals that act on different organs and systems. By varying their consumption, you avoid overloading the body with the same compounds and offer the body a wider range of nutrients. For example, nettle can be used for a diuretic and restorative action, while burdock focuses more on liver purification. Periodic rotation allows the liver, kidneys, and lymphatic system to work in synergy, maintaining an optimal balance in the long term. In addition, this variety reduces the risk of developing intolerances or addictions, allowing the body to receive the active ingredients with maximum efficiency. In this way, rotation becomes a simple yet powerful strategy to maximize the benefits of herbs and support overall well-being.

Contraindications

A safe and responsible approach to detox herbs requires awareness of the possible contraindications and side effects that can arise, especially if the change to an alkaline diet happens too drastically. Abruptly switching to a diet that excludes commonly consumed foods and introduces numerous cleansing herbs can alter the palate and affect motivation, leading some people to feel deprived of their usual flavors and, as a result, to re-enact toxic habits after a short period. For this reason, it is crucial to consider detox herbal supplementation as an integral part of a lifestyle, not a temporary diet, by taking a step-by-step approach that allows the body to adapt sustainably.

It is advisable to start with small doses, carefully monitor your body's reactions, and progressively increase your intake according to your personal tolerance. A smooth transition helps avoid side effects such as electrolyte imbalances or digestive upset, which can result from excess alkalizing substances. In addition, respecting these precautions allows you to keep motivation high over time, integrating the new regime into your daily routine without feeling deprived or constrained, thus transforming a dietary change into a lasting and positive habit. By carefully following precautions and tailoring the route to your needs, you can achieve significant and lasting benefits, reducing the risks of side effects and promoting better overall health.

CONCLUSIONS

Maintaining long-term health with Dr. Sebi's method means considering nutrition and herbal medicine as integrated parts of a holistic lifestyle, in which the alkaline balance of the body and the choice of non-hybridized herbs become essential elements. To start right away, it is helpful to choose at least one purifying herb, such as nettle or burdock, and combine it with an alkalizing meal; organize your pantry with airtight containers, spices, and herbal powders; maintain adequate hydration; experiment with small daily changes, such as replacing an industrial snack with an alkaline smoothie; and keep track of progress, listening to the signals that the body sends. It is precisely in this gradual introduction of new habits that a relationship of harmony with oneself is built, allowing the immune system to work at its best and the self-healing processes to be activated with constancy and depth. You have all the essential information to embark on a wellness path based on Dr. Sebi's principles. Remember that the key to success lies in the constancy and listening of your body: small daily changes can generate profound and lasting transformations over time. We sincerely thank you, the reader, for dedicating your time and attention to this book. Your journey to natural, integrated health starts now: be open to experimenting, learning, and growing, knowing that every step forward is a precious gift you give to yourself. Suppose you found this book helpful and would like to support our work. In that case, we invite you to leave an honest review on Amazon: your contribution will help others discover and embark on the same path of health and awareness. Have a good walk!

Made in the USA
Middletown, DE
21 June 2025